THE
CLEAN
FREAK
MANIFESTO

THE CLEAN FREAK MANIFESTO

THE GERMAPHOBE'S GUIDE TO
Sanitizing Everything in Your Home

TARA D. GARNER

CASTLE POINT
BOOKS

THE CLEAN FREAK MANIFESTO.
Copyright © 2021 by St. Martin's Press. All rights reserved.
Printed in China. For information, address St. Martin's Press, 120 Broadway, New York, NY 10271.

www.castlepointbooks.com

The Castle Point Books trademark is owned by Castle Point Publishing, LLC. Castle Point books are published and distributed by St. Martin's Publishing Group.

ISBN 978-1-250-27660-5 (trade paperback)
ISBN 978-1-250-27577-6 (ebook)

Design by Tara Long
Images used under license by Shutterstock.com

Our books may be purchased in bulk for promotional, educational, or business use. Please contact your local bookseller or the Macmillan Corporate and Premium Sales Department at 1-800-221-7945, extension 5442, or by email at MacmillanSpecialMarkets@macmillan.com.

First Edition: 2021

10 9 8 7 6 5 4 3 2 1

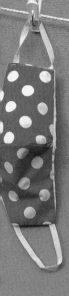

CONTENTS

YOU HAVE THE POWER

Taking Control against Germs

IS YOUR PURSE OR BRIEFCASE CLEANER THAN A TOILET? Chances are, not so much. A recent study found that *more than 95 percent* of men's and women's bags carried bacterial contamination. Researchers say carryalls pick up unsanitary bugs from bathrooms and kitchen tables and are rarely cleaned. As your bags move around your house, car, and office, they become giant mobile germ hot spots. But they're just one super-spreader in our daily lives.

No matter how savvy you think you are about germ control, there are likely at least a few germ hot spots—like your purse, shoes, touchscreens, kitchen sponges, even laundry baskets— you might have overlooked. And that's not surprising, even for clean freaks. Our homes may sparkle and shine with no fingers able to write letters in dust, but invisible threats may still lurk. Our rooms may be filled with fresh scents of lavender candles and lemon essential oils, but those germs are still there—enjoying our home as their home.

With the help of *The Clean Freak Manifesto*, you can show these unwelcome guests the door—or stop them before they even enter. Ready to give the buggers a sanitizing surprise and help your household stay healthy? Let's bring all your disinfecting tools and tricks to the table—and the touchscreens, light switches, doorknobs…!

THE GERM CHALLENGE

What makes germ control most difficult is that you can't see coronavirus, *Salmonella*, *E. coli*, or influenza. But pathogenic, or disease-causing, germs can be alive and thriving on surfaces all around you—in your home and on items you bring inside, from that purse or briefcase to takeout dinner and packages delivered. While you can't eradicate every germ in your environment, you can take simple steps to minimize these carriers of ill health.

In today's germophobic society, the very thought of germs makes some of us stop and think about bolting to the closest place to wash our hands. By this point, having lived through a pandemic, most of us know how to wash our hands properly—wet, lather, scrub (at least 20 seconds, or two "Happy Birthday" run-throughs), rinse. We may be less clear on which surfaces in our homes need disinfectant attention.

In fact, we're often operating on panic-cleaning mode. You hear a news report on the bacteria or virus surface hot spot du jour, grab bleach in hand, follow the moving target to crazy-clean, and decimate your cozy upholstered couch or smart speaker in the process.

Clear Expectations

Let's be realistic: you'll never erase every germ from your house. Do your best and don't stress! The truth is, not all bacteria actually cause us to get sick. And some exposure to germs is actually good for us, medical experts say, as it helps build our immune systems and keeps us healthier in the long run. *Control* is your magic word, and opportunity abounds to do just that.

Now imagine this: you know how to clean and sanitize the stuff you're bringing into your home—mail, groceries, takeout—and the hard and soft items and surfaces already inside. Your plan covers any immediate threat hitting the news headlines—and ones that may come down the road. Cleaning electronics from smartphones to wearable technology will no longer be a mystery. Feeling smart, prepared, and safe, you settle into your safely sanitized sofa and chill.

Your best approach, even if you are the most gung ho of germaphobes: stay calm, understand how germs operate and where they congregate, and form a science-driven plan of attack that works for your real life—all of which this book is designed to help you do. *The Clean Freak Manifesto* covers everything you need to know to keep your home truly clean and healthy amid the ever-changing world of viruses and bacteria. We'll walk through, step by step, how to safely and sanely sanitize your entire home.

Starting with the basic tenets of cleaning and disinfecting that meet current Centers for Disease Control (CDC) standards, we'll move into sanitizing all of the hard and soft surfaces and items throughout our homes. If that sounds overwhelming even for a clean freak, don't worry! You'll find help to prioritize the top spots to hit when available time is tight, plus shortcuts and natural cleaning choices to give lots of effective options that work for your needs.

What if no matter what you do, those sneaky bugs break through and someone in the household gets sick? *The Clean Freak Manifesto* focuses on healthy living and eradicating germs, including measures you can take to keep everyone in the home safe and healthy when a family member is sick. From sanitizing common areas to safe laundry handling, you'll know how to stop the spread of bacteria and viruses.

LET'S START SANITIZING

With all of the information (and disinformation) you can find on battling germs, there is one important point I want you to know from the start. All of the cleaning and sanitizing strategies in these pages are time-tested. I've gleaned them from sources ranging from knowledgeable contacts (both the clean freak and germaphobe variety) to the extensive research I have scoured for my *San Francisco Chronicle* cleaning column "Coming Clean." At the same time, these strategies are also pandemic-perfected, as my usual cleaning routine underwent dramatic changes in the face of new and evolving germs and viruses.

One thing hasn't changed: cleaning and disinfecting are the essential one-two punch for knocking out the germs we can read about in history books and today's nefarious new viruses and bacteria on our home's surfaces. Chapter 1 sets up these two super tools in your healthy living arsenal, so you're ready to dive in to your battle against germs. From there, the sky—or the roof in our homes—is the limit to controlling germs all through your daily spaces.

The fact that you're holding this book lets me know I am not alone in the quest to step up the usual cleaning and disinfecting routine, targeting previously under-the-radar items—like my cell phone, shoes, and deliveries—in addition to the usual cleaning hot spots like the kitchen and bathrooms. We're all in this together as clean freaks and germaphobes, united in a vision for healthier households! The ideas and information in *The Clean Freak Manifesto* can help you make clean living a reality.

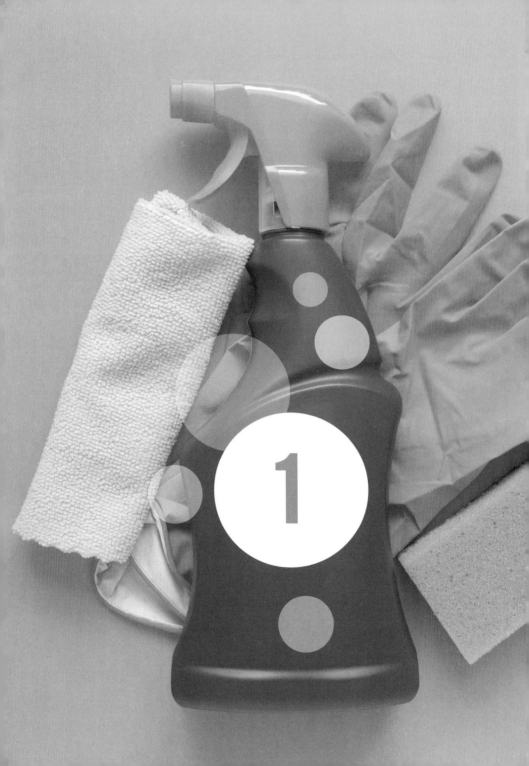

SANITIZING YOUR HOME

Super Starters for Cleaning & Disinfecting

LIVING THROUGH A PANDEMIC has opened our collective eyes to a whole new world of germs out there—one that we're now seemingly called upon to conquer daily at home and wherever our travels take us. Germaphobes everywhere are on high alert, viewing every surface as a potentially lethal petri dish. Properly sanitizing the various items and surfaces in our homes has become the new mandate for healthy living.

The pandemic may have you wanting to scrub down every surface in your home. But before you empty your local store of its entire stock of bleach, it's important to know all of your options for cleaning and disinfecting—and how and where each works best. You're about to get the scoop on how to kick germs out of your home safely and effectively—copious quantities of bleach not required.

THE DISINFECTING DIFFERENCE

Cleaning and disinfecting—especially focusing on the high-touch surfaces in our homes—can slow the spread of pathogenic germs and help keep us healthy. While the two words are often used interchangeably, cleaning and disinfecting are two distinct steps. Together, they are the dream team against germs. What's the difference?

CLEANING removes dirt and *some* germs from surfaces. Simple soap and water is one of the most popular cleaning methods. The cleaning process, however, does not kill germs lurking on a surface. So, why not skip right to disinfecting? Cleaning is a smart start to the two-step process because it lowers germ numbers as well as the risk of spreading infection. Removing surface gunk also gives a follow-up disinfectant the clean surface it requires to do its germ-killing job effectively. Otherwise, dirt and oil could actually consume or trap the disinfectant before it ever reaches the germs.

Easy All-Purpose Cleaning Spray

This homemade cleaning solution works well on hard surfaces. In a spray bottle, gently swirl 2 cups of water, ½ cup of distilled white vinegar, ¼ cup of isopropyl (rubbing) alcohol, and ⅛ teaspoon of dishwashing liquid. To scent, add 5 to 10 drops of essential oil.

DISINFECTING with a household disinfectant is the essential second step that kills 99.9 percent of surface germs (when used according to directions) to further lower the risk of spreading infection. Disinfectants are antimicrobials regulated by the Environmental Protection Agency (EPA). Disinfectants attack microscopic organisms (i.e., bacteria, viruses, and fungi) on surfaces. This process does not always make a dirty surface appear clean. But by killing surface germs after cleaning, it will make your home both look and truly be clean.

SANITIZING is the middle sister of cleaning and disinfecting. Although we use the word *sanitize* casually as another way to imply germ-free, sanitizers are technically cleaning products that lower the germ count to a safer level, per public health standards and requirements. They come in especially handy on the go—when full disinfecting isn't always practical. Sanitizing products do not carry an EPA registration number.

THE BOTTOM LINE: Clean surfaces are not necessarily disinfected, and disinfected surfaces are not necessarily clean. The most effective way to mitigate the spread of bacteria and viruses is to clean an object or surface first and then disinfect it. This diligence is most critical in certain areas of your home.

The biggest threat to you and your family's health and safety are the frequently touched objects and surfaces. Because the more you—and everyone around you—touch a surface, the more germs and bacteria collect on that surface and lie in wait to jump on your hands. The most frequently touched surfaces in most homes are places like tables, chairs, telephones, keyboards, remote controls, countertops, and doorknobs. Because

Germ Face-off

Cleaning and disinfecting high-touch surfaces daily lessens the chance of transmitting germs or viruses that can make us ill when we touch our eyes, nose, or face—as we do on average 12 times an hour, according to one recent study.

these places see so much daily action, they should be disinfected daily to reduce the number of germs waiting there the next time someone flips on a light switch or pulls out a chair for dinner. If you need to prioritize your cleaning time and efforts, science leads us to the areas to focus on—those high-touch hot spots—and how to tackle them efficiently in Chapter 2.

BEST HOUSEHOLD GERM-KILLERS

When killing surface germs is the name of the game, look for cleaning products with disinfectant properties. Cleaning products that say "disinfectant" on the label are required to meet government specifications. To ensure the product has met all government requirements for effectiveness, look for an EPA registration number on the label. Active ingredients may include:

- Sodium hypochlorite (chlorine bleach)
- Hydrogen peroxide
- Isopropyl (rubbing) alcohol
- Ethanol
- Pine oil
- Citric acid
- Quaternary ammonium compounds (i.e., quats)

Bleach, hydrogen peroxide, and rubbing alcohol are good examples of generic products that are proven to disinfect surfaces throughout your home, including tile, bathroom surfaces, walls, and floors. You can also find many disinfectant formulas available under brand names.

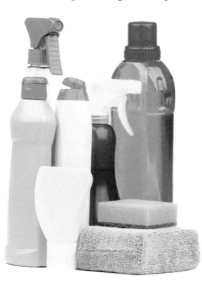

Tested Formulas

Probably the easy way to disinfect and trust the results is to use a proven disinfectant product. Fortunately, you don't need to be a disinfectant detective to find a formula that works. The EPA publishes lists of products it has tested and found to be effective at killing viruses, bacteria, and all kinds of germs.

- Search for "registered disinfectants" at epa.gov. For products to receive registration, a manufacturer must submit lab test results and descriptions of its manufacturing processes to the EPA. The EPA then reviews the data to deem it legit.

- You can also locate the EPA registration number on a product label, then enter the first two sets of numbers into a search tool on epa.gov to find out for which germ-killing claims the particular product has been approved.

- Another option to find EPA registered choices: read a product's label and look for words like *kills germs* or *eliminates bacteria*. Until a manufacturer proves its product kills germs through verified testing, it may not make such public health claims on its label.

Basic Bleach

Chlorine bleach—the kind that's not safe for colors—is a strong economical disinfecting agent that has been used for decades. Look for bleach containing 5.2 to 8.25 percent sodium hypochlorite. But you don't need to—and shouldn't—bathe your surfaces in pure bleach to get beneficial effects. Because bleach is so strong, always dilute it with water.

> ### CLEAN CHOICES
> **2-in-1 Products**
>
> If the surface in question is not visibly dirty, clean it with an EPA-registered product that cleans by removing germs and disinfects by killing the germs. Follow label directions, as there are often different tactics for applying the product as a cleaner versus as a disinfectant.

You will find different bleach-to-water ratios for use with regular bleach, depending on the source. The CDC recommends ⅓ cup of bleach per gallon of water, or 4 teaspoons of bleach per quart of water. Some product labels recommend a slightly stronger ½ cup of bleach per gallon of water, or 2 tablespoons of bleach per quart of water.

The Cleaning Management Institute, a provider of training and certification for professional cleaning services, recommends a still stronger 1:10 ratio (about 1½ cups of bleach per gallon of water, or about ⅓ cup of bleach per quart of water); some medical disinfectants are basically the same solution. You can use your judgment and comfort level to determine what solution is best for what you're cleaning. In most cases throughout *The Clean Freak Manifesto*, we'll follow the CDC.

To make an effective disinfecting solution for colorfast, non-porous surfaces, follow the CDC recipe:

- Mix ⅓ cup of bleach into a gallon of room-temperature or warm water, or 4 teaspoons of bleach per quart of water. Avoid mixing with hot water, which can cause the release of additional chlorine gas into the air.

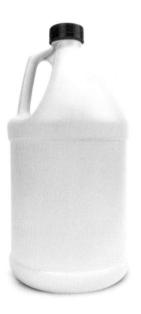

- Sponging the mixture on surfaces is the simplest way to get disinfecting. You can also place the mixture in a spray bottle and spritz liberally on surfaces. Make sure there are no metal parts on your bottle's trigger—bleach corrodes metal, which can introduce rust and contaminate your mixture.

Let the bleach mixture rest on the surface for at least 10 minutes before wiping it off with a soft cleaning cloth. If you don't give a disinfectant enough time to do its work, you're not disinfecting. You're wasting time and product.

Follow instructions for application and these best practices for working with bleach:

- Ensure proper ventilation—simply cracking a window open can help.

- Wear gloves and safety glasses for added protection.

- Don't use a recycled bottle or old mixture. You'll have 24 hours to safely and effectively use a bleach and water solution.

- Keep bleach bottles away from heat and sunlight. When storing, find a cool dry place to store the bleach.

- Toss bleach if it's been more than one year since the product was made. How will you know? Again, the product label is the place to go for all the important information you will need to safely use a product. When looking for an expiration date on the bleach bottle, look for letters and numbers printed on the product label. Be on the lookout for a sequence that looks like this: MR20106. This seemingly random set of letters and numbers means it was made in 2020 on the 106th day of the year. Don't worry about the letters as much as the numbers.

Better Not with Bleach

Bleach is so powerful that there are certain times to pass it by.

- No mixing with ammonia. The combo forms a toxic gas.

- No touching your screen. Bleach will destroy the oleophobic (fingerprint-resistant) coating on your cell phone's screen.

- No mixing with metal. Bleach is corrosive, eating away at metal surfaces.

- No bare wood. Bleach can cause bare wood grains to swell.

- No upholstered furniture. Bleach can leave stains on upholstery.

Places to disinfect with bleach: Countertops, sinks, faucets, tubs, toilets, doorknobs, drawer pulls, light switches, plastic toy boxes, and painted wood furniture, cabinets, and doors.

TRY A CLEANING COCKTAIL

When cleaning tasks are at hand, go ahead and reach for a bottle of vodka. Yes, you read that right. No, it's not happy hour . . . yet.

Shaken or stirred, odorless vodka is a perfect cleaning solution for the chemically sensitive and an excellent degreaser. Although most forms of vodka contain alcohol concentrations too low to be considered an effective disinfectant (around 40 percent versus the minimum 70 percent needed), you can take advantage and use it as an all-purpose cleaner.

So, the next time you need to show that grimy tub ring or crumby countertop who's boss, stir up a "cleaning cocktail." You can use vodka by itself, or create a cleaning solution using a 1:1 vodka-water mix. To use:

- Dip a sponge or rag in the vodka cleaning solution, apply to the surface to be cleaned, and wipe off. You can also put the solution in a spray bottle for easy spritzing and cleaning.

- To keep those unsightly toilet rings from forming, pour a half cup of vodka into the bowl monthly. Let sit overnight, if possible, and flush clean. While you're there, wipe down the seat and lid.

- To add a fresh citrus scent, fill a spray bottle with vodka, drop in some lemon or orange peels, and let it sit. The citric acid in the orange peels will be dissolved by the vodka, further boosting vodka's cleaning might.

No need to break out the top-shelf bottle—the cheap stuff works just as well for less.

Hydrogen Peroxide

According to the CDC, hydrogen peroxide is a safe and effective way to kill bacteria, viruses, and fungi on hard nonporous surfaces. Hydrogen peroxide produces free radicals that attack potential sources of infection and disease. The foaming bubbles you inevitably see when hydrogen peroxide comes into contact with a contaminated object? That's the result of the free radicals going to work for you.

Hydrogen peroxide comes in a variety of strength levels. For use as a disinfectant at home, use the 3 percent hydrogen peroxide found at your local grocery store or pharmacy. It's inexpensive and easy to find. Skip the high-percentage hydrogen peroxide used for hair lightening or labeled as "food grade." At high concentrations, hydrogen peroxide is a powerful bleaching agent, which is the reason it makes hair lighter and can damage household surfaces.

As with every household disinfectant in your arsenal, this product's effectiveness depends on proper use during application. When it comes time to disinfect a surface, always clean it first. You can use hydrogen peroxide right out of the bottle; let sit on the surface for 1 minute before wiping dry.

To get the most benefit from your brown bottle, follow these guidelines:

- Store the bottle in a cool dark place—not your bathroom's medicine cabinet.

- Use hydrogen peroxide before the expiration date and within six months.

Brown Reasoning

Hydrogen peroxide comes in that basic brown bottle for a good reason. Exposure to the light forces the active ingredients in hydrogen peroxide to decompose into water and oxygen, rendering the product utterly ineffective for the purpose at which we are looking. The decomposition destroys the free radicals needed for an effective disinfectant. Always leave hydrogen peroxide in the original bottle, rather than transferring it to a prettier container. You can jazz up your cleaning routine by slipping the bottle into a beverage koozie.

- Not sure if your bottle is still effective? Here's an easy test: Pour a bit into a sink. If it bubbles (reacting with the metal), it's still good as a germ fighter.

When using hydrogen peroxide, test first in an inconspicuous surface area to make sure it doesn't discolor or fade the surface. Hydrogen peroxide is acidic and has bleaching properties, so it won't always be safe to use on every surface and object you want to disinfect. If a surface is prone to bleaching or etching, hydrogen peroxide is not the product you want to use. These surfaces include but are not limited to:

- Marble, granite, and other natural stone (If you must use hydrogen peroxide, always dilute it with equal parts water.)

- Certain metals (e.g., lead, brass, copper, and zinc)

PLACES TO DISINFECT WITH HYDROGEN PEROXIDE: Tubs, tile, and grout; toilets; small metal items, such as keys and tools; wooden cutting boards; refrigerator; sponges (both kitchen and bathing) and makeup blenders; thermometers; razors; and toothbrushes.

Isopropyl (Rubbing) Alcohol

Isopropyl or rubbing alcohol will kill most bacteria and fungi and many viruses; somehow, the norovirus can stand its own against alcohol. However, keep in mind that rubbing alcohol evaporates very quickly. That quick evaporation makes it tough to keep treated surfaces wet for the time necessary to disinfect. Rubbing alcohol is best used on small and hard surfaces. For the best disinfecting results:

- Look for 70 percent alcohol concentration. Know that higher isn't always better. Isopropyl alcohol at 99 percent is pure isopropanol and evaporates before it can attack germs.

- Keep the surface visibly wet for a minimum of 30 seconds to ensure the alcohol destroys all germs.

PLACES TO DISINFECT WITH ALCOHOL: Computer keyboards, remote controls, smartphones, and anything else with a touchscreen. Just don't soak your electronics or get liquid near any openings.

What About Ultraviolet (UV) Light?

Hospitals use ultraviolet light in the form of UVC—the highest-energy category—to disinfect equipment and rooms. Some cities use UV power to disinfect drinking water. So, does it work for us? The verdict is tricky.

Clear testing standards for consumer-oriented UV devices are lacking. So, it's difficult to really know the effectiveness of what you can buy for everyday home use. UVC devices need to operate in a very specific wavelength band to be effective. Manufacturers of home devices have been caught on false claims. Plus, there is real risk for skin and eyes involved with UVC devices, if used improperly.

SANITIZING SURPRISE
The Verdict on Classic Cleaners

Wondering if old standbys work for your modern household's needs? Vinegar cleans glass and kills food germs. Ensure the surface remains wet for at least 10 minutes to eradicate any trace of *Salmonella.* However, vinegar will not be effective against most viruses and bacteria. Baking soda can absorb odor in your fridge and work as a general surface cleaner but not a disinfectant. For cleaning, add 4 tablespoons of baking soda to 1 quart of water, or sprinkle some on a wet sponge.

You can turn to sunlight for easy UV treatment, but it takes some time to have true benefits. In real life, turning to a disinfectant you can apply and wipe off in minutes is likely a more practical proven path.

DIY DISINFECTING WIPES

Disinfecting wipes you can buy in a pop-up canister or pouch are convenient and simple to use, and kill most bacteria and viruses on hard surfaces. These store-bought disinfecting wipes are pricey, however. There's also a sad environmental impact of using disposable wipes. They all come in plastic jugs or packages that add to the landfill or wind up in the ocean unless recycled. As for the wipes themselves, most include polyester or polypropylene materials. These materials aren't biodegradable, so they'll never break down.

Fortunately, you can make disinfecting wipes at home with just a few simple ingredients. These homemade wipes are not only better for your budget. If you use cloth instead of paper products, they're better for the environment, too.

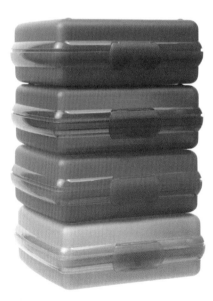

1. Choose the Container

Use a non-metallic container for your wipes. Metal cans or jars will rust, and rusty wipes more or less defeat the purpose. Reusing an old wipes container is one easy idea, or try the following:

- Quart- or gallon-sized jar with a plastic lid
- Glass mason jar
- Plastic cereal storage container
- Other plastic food container

Make sure the lid to your container of choice fits well, so your homemade wipes won't dry out.

2. Choose the Towels

The paper products that you use to make the wipes should be strong enough to stand up to some serious surface cleaning while they are wet. Good choices for the job include:

- Heavy-duty paper towels
- Paper guest hand towels
- Paper napkins (full-size or cut into smaller pieces)

If you prefer more eco-friendly reusable wipes, good material choices include:

- 100 percent cotton cloths
- Bamboo cloth
- Microfiber washcloths

Reusable wipes should be machine washed in hot water after every use.

3. Layer the Towels

Separate the towels into individual pieces and fold or roll to fit your container. If you are reusing a pop-up wipe container, fold them with one layer interwoven with the next towel so they will pull up together. If you have a round container, cut a roll of paper towels in half, and remove the inner cardboard core to create a pull-from-the-center roll of wipes.

4. Measure the Alcohol and Essential Oils

In a separate container, pour enough isopropyl alcohol (70 percent or higher) to cover and saturate the towels. Three cups of alcohol will saturate about 40 folded paper towels.

Your Germ-Fighting Solution

Look for isopropyl alcohol—sold in drug and grocery stores—in a 70 percent solution. Using less than 70 percent alcohol will not provide the microbe-killing protection you desire.

Next, add 10 to 20 drops of essential oils to the alcohol, if desired. Essential oils add a pleasant scent, and some oils do have antibacterial qualities. Recommended oils with some anti-bacterial qualities include tea tree, lavender, geranium, lemon, orange, eucalyptus, rosemary, cinnamon, clove, thyme, and peppermint oils.

5. Saturate and Cover the Wipes

Pour about half of the alcohol (mixed with essential oils, if using) over the towels. Wait until the liquid is absorbed, then pour in the rest. You might need to add a bit more alcohol if the towels are not fully soaked. Some liquid should be visible in the container. Cover the container tightly. The wipes are now ready for disinfecting action whenever you need them!

STEPS FOR EFFECTIVE DISINFECTING

It's not just *what* you use to clean and disinfect; it's also *how* you clean and disinfect.

1. Get Gloved

Gloves help keep germs off your hands as you clean while also protecting your skin from harsh products. Toss disposable rubber, vinyl, or latex gloves after using, so you don't spread any illness-causing viruses or bacteria. If you prefer reusable gloves, dedicate a pair to disinfecting and wash them thoroughly afterward. Whatever type of gloves you wear, don't forget to wash your hands after you remove them. Germs can be sneaky, and glove removal gives them opportunity for transferral—no matter how careful you are.

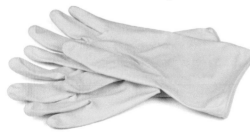

2. Clean the Surface First

Ensure the surface is washed with soap and water or an all-purpose cleaner. Remember: your disinfectant works better when the surface is clearer at the start. Plus, your surfaces will be shiny-clean and germ-free.

Required Reading

It takes just a minute to read directions on the label of any cleaner or disinfectant you're using. Check the recommended "use sites" and "surface types" to see what's safe and effective. Watch for warnings about mixing with other products and any other precautionary statements.

3. Don't Rush the Process

It may be tempting to squirt and wipe in a record-setting attempt. But disinfection is not instantaneous—no matter what you wished on your 2020 birthday candle. You only are wasting your time and products (and, in turn, money) if you don't allow the disinfectant to take the time it needs to work. Let disinfectants sit on the surface you're cleaning for the label-prescribed time before wiping clean. The surface should remain visibly wet throughout the process—do not allow it to dry.

4. Know When to Rinse

When disinfecting surfaces that come into contact with food items (such as kitchen counters and cutting boards), rinse them with water after the disinfectant dries to ensure a safe surface for future use with food.

5. Watch for Germ Hitchhikers

It's easy to carry germs from the bathroom to the kitchen via a shared cleaning cloth or sponge. Using a different color sponge or cloth for each room can help you keep them straight.

It's best to launder cleaning rags immediately. Use a long wash cycle, hot water, and add a laundry sanitizer like bleach to the wash water. Dry your cleaning rags in a hot dryer for a minimum of 45 minutes, or line dry them in bright sunlight for added disinfection. If you've tossed cleaning rags into a hamper or laundry basket, be sure to clean and disinfect it after starting the wash to avoid cross-contamination. To clean sponges, soak them in a 1:10 diluted bleach solution.

6. Keep Everything Secure

Always store cleaners and disinfectants in their original containers with the lids tightly closed. Clearly label and date any mixtures you make at home in a spray bottle to avoid confusion and expired cleaners, and to ensure an overall safe cleaning environment.

It's best to keep all of your cleaning products together in a temperature-controlled area inside your home—ideally it should be a clean, cool, and dry place like a cabinet, so the chemicals are not exposed to the elements. Keep your germ-fighting arsenal below eye level (not on a high shelf) to avoid falling bottles and spills, but also to store cleaners and disinfectants out of the reach of curious little hands and inspecting pet noses. Safety locks are a smart addition to any cabinets or drawers that contain disinfectants, to avoid accidental ingestion by children or pets.

Now you're equipped with powerful cleaning and disinfecting knowledge. Where to start kicking some germs out the door? Let Chapter 2 guide you to your home's germ hot spots.

CLEAN UP YOUR CLEANING STORAGE

Cleanups are much more manageable when tools and supplies are readily accessible. Stock up on the essentials—brooms, mops, scrubbers, cleaners, rags, and paper towels—then store them strategically. Here are some simple suggestions:

CARRY A SUPPLY CADDY. A supply caddy makes it easy to tote your cleaning stash from room to room. When you have a moment to clean, just pick up and go. Consider creating two caddies—one for the kitchen and bath, and another for living areas. Fill each with room-specific cleaning supplies.

GO VERTICAL. Wooden pegs affixed to a wall in a utility area can keep bulky cleaning tools like mops and brooms together while maximizing space. A hanging net bag is a handy place to store partially damp rags or sponges. Later, use it to haul them to the washing machine.

BOX IT UP. Lidded plastic boxes organize buffing cloths and other small items that could get lost or jumbled on a cabinet shelf. These boxes should be easy to carry where they're needed.

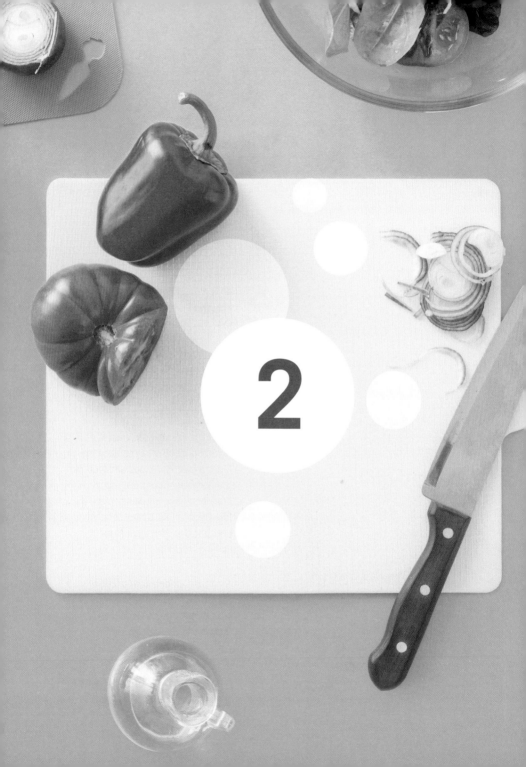

2

HIGH-TOUCH HOT SPOTS

What to Hit Daily, Weekly & Monthly

THE HOME MAY BE WHERE THE HEART IS, but it is also where bacteria and viruses set up shop. These nasty little interlopers thrive even in households that look brilliantly clean. They ride home from school on your child's hands, stow away on your handbag or briefcase, enter with foods that you bring home, and grow and multiply around the sink.

Keeping household germs at bay is essential if we're going to prevent colds, flu, and other infectious illnesses from spreading. If left unchecked, these unwelcome tagalongs can cause illnesses ranging from the common cold and stomach bugs to food poisoning and COVID-19.

Not all germs are harmful, thankfully. But where there are germ strongholds, the conditions are favorable for disease-causing viruses and bacteria to lurk. Things like the flu or respiratory syncytial virus (RSV) can linger 6 to 24 hours on hard surfaces, while bacteria like *Salmonella* and *Campylobacter* (i.e., foodborne illnesses) stick around 1 to 4 hours. Just think about how much opportunity for contact with a virus there is in a 24-hour period!

Don't get bogged down by the germ numbers. Although, at times, it can seem that germs have the advantage—they can be seemingly everywhere at once. You? Not so much. Nonetheless, you can win the battle against household germs. You have the upper hand, after all!

Although you really can't eliminate germs entirely, some simple housekeeping steps go a long way toward keeping harmful bugs at bay. By focusing your cleaning and disinfecting efforts on the significant germ hot spots, you'll be able to keep things well under control to ensure that your family has a much better shot at staying well.

UNCOVERING WHERE GERMS LURK

You can't see them, so how can you beat them? You must know where the germiest bugs lurk, and how to zap them. Among clean freaks everywhere, these germy spots in our homes are known as "high-touch areas" and require frequent disinfection to reduce illness transmission within our homes.

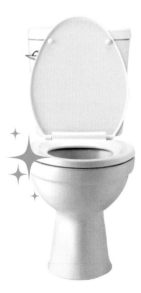

Your gut might lead you to believe that most of these hot spots are in your home's bathrooms. While bathrooms do shelter their share of germs, the biggest problem spot is actually the kitchen. That seemingly clean place where we prep and cook food has been uncovered as one of the most germ-laden areas of the home. In fact, according to some studies, you'd do better to eat off the toilet. Researchers at the University of Arizona studied 14 areas in the kitchen and bath for germ count. The top five germiest areas were in the kitchen: sponges and dishcloths, the sink drain area, the sink faucet handle, cutting boards, and the refrigerator handle. Ready for this? The toilet seat came up *dead last* on the germ scale.

In areas all across the house, light switches, phones, remote controls, and doorknobs are also favorite spots for any of the 150 sneeze- and cough-creating common viruses today, and the lesser-known but equally unpleasant rotavirus, which causes diarrhea, especially in infants. These bugs can survive for hours on hard home surfaces, especially plastic and metals, and children's and pets' toys.

Knowing what you're up against, are you worried that it's time to throw in the towel? No way! You're too tough and committed to the clean cause for that. A smart plan of attack is all you need to maximize your germ control while minimizing your effort and time investment.

THE DIRTY DOZEN TO CLEAN DAILY

By focusing your daily cleaning efforts on your home's high-touch surfaces, you can reduce the transmission of all sorts of potentially contagious bacteria and viruses between family members. Even if you don't have a lot of time to spend cleaning, you can do it right—and fast. Most of these germ hits take just a few minutes, and some can be accomplished while multitasking. Here's how to attack the hot spots.

1. Clean Those Screens

Your phone and other touchscreens deserve some daily disinfecting attention. Give them a good refresh with a disinfecting wipe as you pick them up in the morning and then again every time you return after

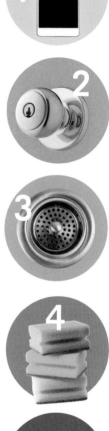

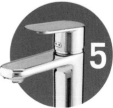

leaving the house. It takes just a minute for a high ROI in the fight against nasty germs. Don't forget the cases that face the front lines of germs just as much as the devices! Remember, you can save both money and environmental impact by making your own disinfecting wipes. Get the step-by-step instructions in Chapter 1 (page 18).

2. Disinfect Doorknobs

Focus on heavily used doorknobs (think: exterior and bathroom doors!) for daily cleaning. Your handiest tool of attack against germs on these tricky surfaces: a disinfecting wipe helps to cover the surface.

3. Send Sink Germs Down the Drain

Even with good handwashing, sinks are super germy spots. To treat them to a daily disinfectant bath, fill the sink with a basic disinfecting solution (⅓ cup of bleach in 1 gallon of warm water). Keep the sink full for 10 minutes, then let the bleachy water (and all the nasties) run down the drain. In just one simple step, you've sanitized the sink and the drain! Time it for the end of the day after rinsing or washing any dishes, and enjoy some sips of tea or wine while you drown the germs. It's downright cathartic.

SANITIZING SURPRISE
Your Microwave's Power

The test: sponges and scrubbing pads were soaked in wastewater containing a mix of fecal bacteria, *E. coli*, and bacterial spores, then microwaved on full power for 2 minutes. The results: more than 99 percent of all the germs and the bacterial spores in the sponges and pads were killed or inactivated, according to a study published in the *Journal of Environmental Health*.

4. Zap Germs from Sponges

While your sink is enjoying that sanitizing soak, whisk any sponges and plastic scrubbers away to a warmer climate to shed germs. The microwave is a perfect sanitizing locale for sponges and plastic scrubbers. To give them the best break from germs, zap those cleaning tools for a full 2 minutes. To do this safely, only microwave sponges or plastic scrubbers without steel or other metals, and make sure the sponge or scrubber is wet, not dry. Two minutes in the microwave should be enough to kill most disease-causing germs. Be careful when removing the sponge, as it will be hot and should not be handled immediately. Another option: soak sponges in a 1:10 diluted bleach solution.

5. Hit Those Handles

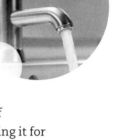

How many times do hands open the fridge, freezer, microwave, and oven in your house? Turn sink faucets on and off? Disinfect appliance and faucet handles daily with a disposable disinfecting wipe or spray them with a combination cleaner/disinfectant. To make your own cheap effective disinfectant, simply mix 4 teaspoons of bleach per quart of water. Apply it to the surface, saturating it for 2 minutes. That's it—no rinsing. Allow to air-dry. Treat frequently used cabinet and drawer handles in the kitchen and bathrooms, too. The germs on those handles have been handled!

6. Sweep Kitchen Central

From serving as a sandwich-making station to sorting mail, kitchen countertops see a lot of action—and can shelter a lot of germs. Clean and disinfect counter surfaces frequently, particularly before and after preparing a meal or snack, with a disinfecting wipe or spray. Check the manufacturer's directions for specialty countertops.

7. Freshen Cutting Boards

They're some of the hardest-working tools in the kitchen, so make sure they're ready for a fresh start after every use. Generally, all it takes is washing with hot water and dish soap, with extra scrubbing given to any places where the board has marks.

If you've been working with meat or poultry, step up your cleaning with a mixture of 4 teaspoons of liquid bleach and 1 quart of water. Apply the mixture to the surface of either your wooden or plastic cutting board, keeping it wet for 10 minutes. Rinse well and let dry. Bonus: the treatment will chase away tough stains and odors as well as bacteria. For a bleach-free option: soak your board in a mixture of 1 part white vinegar to 4 parts water for a few minutes, then rinse well and let dry. Ready for your next fabulous food adventure!

8. Tackle That Toilet

Disinfect the handles, lids, and seats—germy strongholds—at least once a day with a spray or wipe, and several times a day if someone in your home is ill.

9. Swipe Light Switches

Shut off the spreading power of germs by disinfecting those switches and switch plates at least daily. Boost your approach to more than once a day when the flu or another virus is circulating. Hit these spots easily with disinfectant wipes, or follow the label instructions on a spray disinfectant.

10. Attack Remotes and Game Controllers

To stop germs in their quest to spread, disinfect these high-touch items daily using a wipe or spray. It's a simple game plan to thwart the nasties. If someone in your home is sick, put the remote in a resealable plastic bag and wipe that with a disinfecting wipe several times each day. It's easier to thoroughly wipe the bag's flat surface than get into all the crevices of buttons. Replace the bag at the end of the day.

11. Clear the Table

Kitchen or dining tables may serve as home base for family dinners, but they're often also temporary landing spots for purses or backpacks—after they've been on the floor in a public setting. Disinfect your table before and after meals especially, but also try to target it before any time someone spreads out there to do work or schoolwork. Clean first with a soapy microfiber cloth to remove surface grime, then saturate the surface with a store-bought or homemade disinfectant spray (see #5). Wait 10 minutes for the bleach-based spray to do its work or check the label for brand products, then wipe clean. Check the manufacturer's directions for specialty tables.

12. Don't Forget High-Traffic Chairs

Hard-backed chairs often fly under the radar when you're cleaning. Make sure to disinfect chairs used frequently, including the backs that are touched by hands to pull the chairs out or in. Clean with a quick spritz of disinfectant or a disposable disinfecting wipe.

Doing a daily cleaning and sanitizing sweep of your home's high-touch hot spots makes weekly and deeper monthly cleaning for germ control easier and faster. It rewards you now *and* later!

CLEAN FREAK DAILY CHEAT SHEET

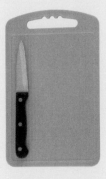

- Phone and touchscreens
- Heavily used doorknobs
- Kitchen sink
- Kitchen sponge/scrubber
- Heavily used handles (appliances, faucets, cabinets, drawers)
- Kitchen countertops and stovetops

- Used cutting boards
- Toilets (handles, lids, seats)
- Light switches
- Remotes and controllers
- Dining tables
- High-traffic hard-backed chairs

HOW TO COME CLEAN SAFELY

If we regularly keep the surfaces that are repetitively touched throughout the day disinfected and clean, then there is less chance of transmitting germs or viruses if we accidentally touch our eyes, nose, or face—as we so often do. Ready to get started cleaning and disinfecting the dirty dozen high-touch surfaces in your home? Start by washing surfaces with an all-purpose household cleaner to remove germs. Rinse and follow with a disinfectant cleaner to kill germs. (In the case of electronics, use an alcohol wipe first to clean, and then a second one to disinfect.)

If you don't have a disinfecting cleaner, make your own bleach disinfecting solution:

- Mix 4 teaspoons of bleach in 1 quart of warm or room-temperature water.

- Don your cleaning gloves, dip a microfiber cloth into the solution, and apply to your surface until it is visibly wet. Let sit for 10 minutes.

- Rinse the solution from the surface with clean water.

If you're using a ready-to-go product, make sure to read the product label directions carefully. Often, there are different methods for using a product as a cleaner and as a disinfectant. Disinfection usually requires the cleaner to remain on the surface for a specific amount of time.

Follow these precautions during your daily disinfecting routine:

- Wearing disposable rubber, vinyl, or latex gloves and changing them between rooms is the best way to prevent germs. Gloves will also protect your hands from strong cleaning products. Toss them when you're done, and always wash your hands thoroughly afterward.

- Always read and follow instructions on a product's label to ensure you have the correct concentration and that it's safe for the surface. Some cleaners can damage surfaces, and if so, the label will provide this information.

- For safety's sake, do not combine cleaning products. Combining some everyday household cleaning products can create dangerous fumes.

- When you're using stronger cleaners or disinfectants—you know, the kind everyone in the house can smell after one spray—do yourself a favor and open a window or three. Adequate ventilation helps the noxious odors show themselves out.

Out the Window

Show airborne germs and allergens the exit by regularly opening your home's windows. Ventilation enables germs to dissipate. In addition, diminishing humidity discourages mold growth.

- Always wash cleaning cloths or rags after you've finished using them in hot water with bleach or another sanitizing laundry additive. Dry the rags in a hot dryer for 45 minutes or line dry them in bright sunlight for added disinfection.

Now that you have an idea of the tasks at hand, here is an efficient way of going about it. Tackle and clean various areas by grouping them (e.g., all doorknobs, all handles, all light switches) and cleaning your way around a room from top to bottom.

WEEKLY SPEED-CLEANING FOR GERMS

Doing a daily cleaning and disinfecting sweep of your home's high-touch hot spots makes weekly cleaning for germ control faster and easier. A cleaner-disinfectant saves time because it combines the two steps—just make sure to read the label for the correct way to do this. The solution will come in handy for cleaning kitchen countertops and bathroom surfaces.

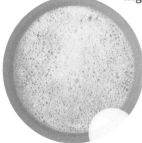

Or you can battle the germs the time-tested way by first cleaning sticky spots or areas in the kitchen and bathroom with warm soapy water (dishwashing liquid works here) to get rid of surface grime before disinfecting. Make your inexpensive disinfecting solution by adding 4 teaspoons of bleach to a quart of water. Wearing gloves to protect your hands, dip a microfiber cloth in the solution, and apply to surfaces until they are visibly wet. Let sit for 10 minutes. Rinse and dry with a clean cloth, or let the surface air-dry.

Even if you don't have a lot of time to spend cleaning, you can do it right—and fast. Once a week, follow these steps to wipe out germs that have set up shop in your home.

Clean Countertops

We give the main countertops attention each day, but there are likely spaces we neglect in the daily rush. Each week, perform a more thorough countertop cleaning. Take everything off your counters and wipe them down with a nonabrasive all-purpose cleaner and disinfectant. Let the counters dry, then put everything back. Check the manufacturer's directions for specialty countertops.

Freshen the Refrigerator

Check for any spills that need cleanup and toss out bad food to keep bacteria from growing. Every few weeks, do a more thorough cleaning.

Clean the Coffee Maker

Clean the coffeepot and filter with a soapy water soak. Wipe down the coffee maker's exterior with a disinfecting wipe.

Hit the Microwave

Treat the interior and exterior to an all-purpose cleaner and disinfectant, according to label directions. Don't forget the keypad. Take out the turntable and wash with dish soap and water, or stick it in the dishwasher if it's dishwasher safe.

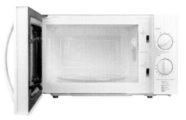

Remove and Wash the Stove Knobs

Those controls see a lot of grime and germ action from splattered foods and food-prepping hands. Hand-wash the knobs or fill the sink with hot soapy water to soak them in for 15 to 20 minutes.

Change Out and Wash Kitchen Dishcloths

Kitchen towels, like kitchen sponges, are a haven for germs. To prevent the spread of germs, change out your kitchen dish towels at least once a week. Wash towels in the washing machine, using hot water, and dry on high heat. Make sure the towels are completely dry before using them. Most bacteria thrive in moisture.

Clean and Disinfect Bathroom Sinks, Tubs, and Toilets

You can save time by spraying cleaners on areas that will benefit from some extra soaking time—like the toilet and tub or shower—and tackling other surfaces while the cleaners do their stuff.

Round Up Bathroom Towels and Bed Linens

Take care not to fluff or shake them, so you don't spread germs and dust around the house. And don't just scoop them up in your arms: it's best to gather them in a laundry basket that you can clean and disinfect after starting the wash to avoid cross-contamination. Wash towels and linens in the warmest water safe for the fabrics.

Pay Attention to Those Toothbrush Holders

Wash or soak all toothbrush holders in warm soapy water, then allow to air-dry. Wipe the toothbrush holder surface with a disinfecting wipe, or place in the dishwasher, on the top rack, if dishwasher safe.

Mop the Floors and Vacuum Carpets

Floors may be more important than you first think when it comes to germ risk. Our kids play on the floor, and we may snuggle with our pets there as well. We set our bags on the floor, which we then move all over the house. It's worth tackling the germs that may be harboring down low. See Chapter 3 (starting on page 46) for the best ways to clean and disinfect hard-surface flooring and Chapter 4 (starting on page 66) for tips on sanitizing carpets.

Give Computer Keyboards Some Love

First, always make sure to turn computers and components off before cleaning. Turn the keyboard upside down, then lightly tap the bottom of the keyboard to dislodge crumbs. Turn back over, and vacuum with a brush attachment. You can also use a can of compressed air to blow the bits out. Go over the keys with a disinfecting wipe that doesn't contain bleach, squeezing first to remove excess moisture. Allow to air-dry.

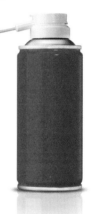

CLEAN FREAK WEEKLY CHEAT SHEET

- Countertops (thorough)
- Refrigerator
- Coffee maker
- Microwave
- Stove knobs
- Kitchen dishcloths
- Bathroom sinks

- Tubs
- Toilets
- Bathroom towels
- Bed linens
- Toothbrush holders
- Floors and carpets
- Computer keyboards

MONTHLY SPEED-CLEANING FOR GERMS

These monthly cleaning chores hardly take any time, and will reward you with a cleaner, healthier home.

Dig into the Refrigerator

Do a more thorough cleaning of the refrigerator interior and toss out old food from the fridge and freezer. For safety, start by unplugging your fridge, then remove all food. As you're taking out items, check expiration dates on all food and condiments inside. Wash all interior surfaces with warm soapy water, then disinfect with a solution of 4 teaspoons of bleach in 1 quart of water. Pay special attention to corners and crevices. Next, rinse the cleaned surfaces with water and dry with a microfiber cloth. Be sure to plug the refrigerator back in! As you return food to the shelving and drawers, place the oldest items that should be used soon front and center for when big and little hands are searching.

Sanitize That Strainer

Put the kitchen sink strainer in the dishwasher to clean and disinfect.

Clean and Disinfect Indoor Trash Cans

Wearing gloves, fill the trash can with hot soapy water and scrub away any spills and drips with a long-handled brush. Rinse and dry, then wipe down the interior with disinfecting wipes.

Clear the Coffee Maker

About once a month, pour in a cup of water and a cup of white vinegar and run it through a brew cycle to deep clean the coffee maker's innards. Then run three or four cycles with water to rinse clean. You could buy a commercial cleaner that does the same thing. But why?

Safeguard Children's and Pets' Toys

Plastic toys are easy. Use soap and water to clean. To disinfect, soak hard plastic toys for 10 minutes in a fresh bleach solution (use ⅓ cup of bleach to 1 gallon of water), rinse, and allow to air-dry. You can also toss plastic toys in the dishwasher on the top shelf—if they don't have batteries. Send plush toys for a hot-water spin in the washing machine, then tumble dry low. Read and follow care labels for instructions (if available).

Sanitize the Washing Machine

Give it a good bath to thank it for all the hard work it does to keep your clothing clean. See Chapter 6 (starting on page 118) for cleaning and disinfecting strategies.

Go Beyond Sheets

While you want to wash bed linens once a week in the hottest water safe for your sheets, your comforter, blanket, and pillows should be washed at least monthly.

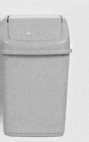

CLEAN FREAK MONTHLY CHEAT SHEET

- Refrigerator (thorough)
- Sink strainer
- Trash cans
- Coffee maker (thorough)
- Kids' and pets' toys
- Washing machine
- Comforters, blankets, and pillows

ROOM BY ROOM

When you're thinking of how you can make the most impact on germs, you might want to think about the places where you and your family spend the most time in your house. It's just another way to consider where germ hot zones are likely to be. Flu viruses can live on some surfaces for a full 24 hours. Norovirus, a common cause of unpleasant intestinal and stomach bugs, will linger even longer, sometimes for days or weeks. Both are excessively contagious. Effectively destroying these left-behind germs will slow or stop the spread of sickness in your home.

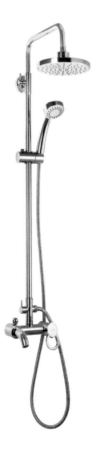

Start Here: The Bathroom

When a family member is sick, the bathroom is even more of a hot spot for spreadable germs. If you think a bug has penetrated your home, start your home cleaning by disinfecting in here.

- Treat hot spots with a mixture of hot water and bleach. Pay attention to the toilet lever, shower faucets, cabinet handles, doorknobs, and light switches.

- To fight mildew in the shower, clean stalls and bathtubs using a nonabrasive, all-purpose disinfectant (antibacterial) cleaner. Always check the product label to see if the product kills germs and mildew, and follow label directions for best results.

- Clean vinyl or ceramic tile using a floor cleaner or a nonabrasive all-purpose cleaner.

Invisible Threats: Kitchen Culprits

The bad news: the kitchen often registers as the germiest room in the house. The good news: proper food handling of items like raw meat, fish, and poultry stops most bacteria associated with them from multiplying to levels that can make you and your family ill.

You can come down with food poisoning as early as 20 minutes and as late as six weeks after consuming your contaminated meal. Always keep in mind the last thing you eat isn't always the culprit when you get sick. The first step in avoiding foodborne illness is easy: take this seriously; it's more common than you might realize. Foodborne illnesses send about 128,000 people to the hospital every year, and you don't want to be one of them. Some of the simplest but most powerful prevention measures follow.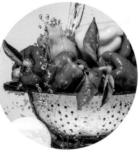

WASH YOUR HANDS AND SURFACES REGULARLY. The most important thing you, as a consumer, can do to ensure your health and safety is the same thing we've been encouraged to do many times—wash your hands with soap and water for at least 20 seconds before and after preparing food.

Washing your hands properly can help prevent the spreading of meat-, poultry-, and fish-borne bacteria onto refrigerator doors, cabinet handles, and countertops, where they'll be ready to infect the next time you return to your refrigerator for a leftover pizza slice from the night before.

When grilling, never serve meat on the same tray or plate used to carry it outside before cooking. If the kitchen counter comes into contact with any uncooked meat, poultry, or fish, grab a few paper towels and clean up the area with hot soapy water.

You can prevent cross-contamination by washing all of the utensils used to prepare raw food in hot soapy water before they are used again. This includes, but is not limited to, every knife, cutting board, and food prep surface that has touched any amount of raw meat, fish, and poultry.

WATCH TEMPERATURES. This one may seem obvious, but don't allow the temperature of your foods to fluctuate too much.

You can't and won't see or smell bacteria and viruses the same way you can see or smell spoiled food. Most of the pathogens found in uncooked foods are killed by cooking the item to an internal temperature of 145°F for roasts or chops of beef, veal, or lamb. Food items such as ground beef and pork need to reach 160°F to consume safely. Cook chicken to 180°F.

BE DEVOTED TO DISINFECTING. To rid your kitchen utensils and surfaces of all germs, you'll need to clean the surface with a diluted bleach solution or a store-bought disinfectant. Keep kitchen surfaces dry when not in use; bacteria survive less than a few hours when moisture is eliminated from the surface.

Sponges and dishcloths—the very things that are supposed to help you destroy lurking germs—can be part of the problem unless you clean them regularly. And, the kitchen towel isn't much better. You don't only use your kitchen towel to dry your

WHEN TO WASH, WHEN *NOT* TO WASH

Every year, roughly one million Americans become sick after eating a contaminated chicken product. Like every animal, chickens have bacteria in their gut to help them digest food. Pathogens like *Campylobacter* and *Salmonella* often contaminate the meat during the packing process, and find their way onto the cutting board and utensils in your kitchen before entering your body. Never wash raw chicken before cooking because it can contaminate your kitchen. Cooking it to an internal temperature of 180°F kills all of the bacteria in chicken.

Unfortunately, many germs can spread long before you pop the entrée inside your oven. *E. coli*, hepatitis A, and *Salmonella*—the most common kitchen contaminants—can find their way onto a sponge or dishcloth; you, in turn, will then spread the bacteria all over your kitchen unless you make an effort to stop them in their tracks.

Yearly, about 1.35 million people in the U.S. contract *Salmonella* poisoning. Infections are most common in summer months when we're consuming watermelon, cantaloupe, and honeydew melon. The vines of these foods grow on the ground, where the rinds often pick up germs. Washed whole melons are best, and make sure to rinse the exterior before slicing open. Refrigerate precut fruits or pack them in ice.

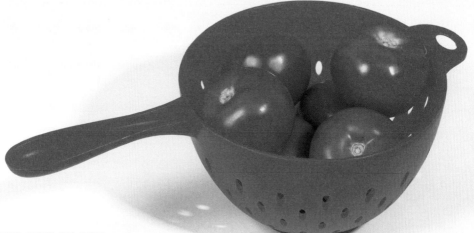

dishes and hands. You use the kitchen towel to clean off grimy little hands and faces, or to wipe up spills on dirty counters. The result: your dish towel can quickly become home to nasty little germs and bugs like *Salmonella* or fecal bacteria. You should replace sponges every few weeks to ensure a sanitary environment. (See page 85 for sponge-disinfecting details.) Regularly toss dishcloths and towels in the washing machine—and always use hot water and bleach.

Dust Away: Bedroom Bliss

Your bed is a cozy nest for dust and dust mites to settle into, too. These allergy triggers lie in wait in sheets, blankets, pillows, carpets, and rugs, and on drapes and blinds. While they are impossible to obliterate, they're harmless unless you have allergies. Still, you might rest more comfortably if you take a few steps to keep these microscopic interlopers in check.

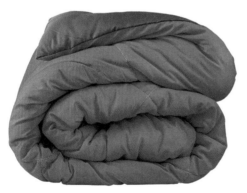

- Wash bed linens once a week in the hottest water safe for your sheets. Your comforter, blanket, and pillows should be washed at least monthly.

- Damp-wipe or vacuum your blinds regularly—they're a virtual magnet for dust.

- Vacuum at least weekly. This simple but powerful step will help keep your home's allergen count down to livable levels. The most useful tool in your cleaning arsenal in the fight against allergens is a vacuum cleaner with a high-efficiency particle air (HEPA) filter. While a HEPA vacuum is ideal, you can find HEPA filters to fit most non-HEPA filtered vacuums these days.

We've taken a tour of the places to concentrate your cleaning and disinfecting efforts. Now, let's see how tackling those high-touch hard surfaces of all kinds throughout your home doesn't need to be hard work. You've made it to Chapter 3!

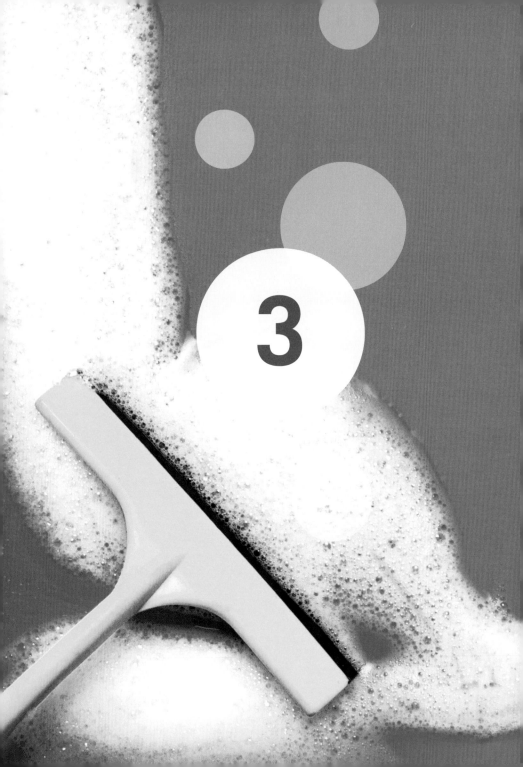

3

TARGETING HARD SURFACES

How to Clean & Disinfect Glass, Metal, Plastic & More

IF YOU CRINGE AT THE THOUGHT of tackling the mildew in the shower or cleaning the grimy refrigerator shelves, you have a lot of company. Many people have mild tendencies this way.

The squeaky-clean truth is that in a sometimes germophobic society, many of us would prefer to do just about anything rather than battle the bacteria, fungi, and viruses around the home. If you're one of them, it may help to keep in mind that there has yet to be an epidemic arising from shoddy housekeeping. That said, most households could still probably afford to step up their game in the disinfecting and sanitizing department without the danger of going to extremes.

It's all about risk mitigation. You can't eliminate risk, but you can often minimize it, and when you do that, you're stacking the odds of staying healthy in your favor.

We're all drawn to the clean we can "see." But we—especially the germaphobes among us—know that just because something looks clean doesn't mean it actually *is* clean. You can't see germs like *Salmonella*, *E. coli*, or influenza. But "pathogenic," or disease-causing, germs like these can be alive and thriving on the hard surfaces all around your home.

So, it just makes sense to minimize the dangers posed by these invisible interlopers. And, your stepped-up efforts to rid your home's glass, metal, plastic, and other hard surfaces of these pesky germs are likely to be well worth the effort.

BEYOND SHINE TO ATTACK GERMS

A recent study found that the SARS-CoV-2 virus, which causes COVID-19, can cling to stainless steel and plastic surfaces for up to 72 hours, much longer than initially thought. Knowing this, it's logical to conclude that glass is an equally germ-drenched surface, likely in dire need of some serious sanitizing.

Even if your surfaces are the shiniest on the block, they can still harbor tons of germs. The glass cleaner you probably have at home may do a killer job on windows, but on germs? Not so much. It's a cleaner, to be sure, but one without disinfecting properties. That means you might be sending surface germs on glass for a swim, but you'd better cross your fingers and hope they drown.

You'll need disinfecting power to really knock out pathogenic, or disease-causing, germs thriving on glass and beyond. To make your home as safe as possible from bacteria and viruses that cause people to be sick, you need to regularly clean and disinfect hard surfaces.

CLEAN CHOICES
Where to Focus Cleaning

Pay serious attention to hard surfaces in your home. In a study by the U.S. National Institutes of Health (NIH), researchers found that the virus that causes COVID-19 can live up to 4 hours on copper, up to 24 hours on cardboard, and up to three days on stainless steel and plastic surfaces.

So, what's the best strategy to truly attack and kill germs on hard nonporous surfaces in your home? Tackle kitchen surfaces, countertops, tables and chairs, sinks, toilets, railings, light switch plates, doorknobs, and metal and plastic toys with these simple but powerful steps.

1. Clean the Hard Surface

Soap and water are all you need. You'll get a great start and set up your disinfectant to go to work when you first remove visible dirt and grime.

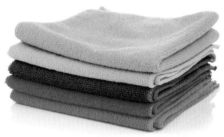

2. Rinse the Surface

Then wipe dry with a clean cloth.

3. Apply a Disinfectant

You can turn to store-bought or make your own (with ⅓ cup of bleach added to 1 gallon of water). Before using, check the disinfectant's label for recommended surfaces. With homemade solutions, test a small amount in an inconspicuous place when using on a surface for the first time.

Put on your cleaning gloves and then apply the solution to the surface using a microfiber cloth or rag. To effectively kill germs, make sure the surface stays wet with the disinfectant for at least 10 minutes, or as instructed on the product label.

4. Rinse and Allow to Air-dry

Rinsing with water is especially crucial on surfaces used to prepare food.

GLASS: IMPROVE YOUR OUTLOOK

Just about any cleaner and disinfectant are safe to use on glass because glass is chemically inert. However, you need to be careful with other transparent plastic materials like polycarbonate and plexiglass because many cleaners cause surface clouding.

When it comes time to clean your plexiglass, your best bet is to use a product specially formulated for the material. (Check with the manufacturer for recommendations.) You can also use soap and water, which will in most cases render germs and viruses less effective or kill at least some portion.

If you want to clean off the fingerprints on your front door, you can stick with the glass cleaner you already have on hand. But if your goal is to clean and disinfect, then you will need to read product labels carefully. Look for cleaners that contain disinfecting ingredients like these:

- L-Lactic acid
- Quaternary ammonium
- Sodium hypochlorite

Here's how to get your home's glass surfaces—including windows, tabletops, and mirrors—smudge-free and, more importantly, germ-free.

1. Clear Away Surface Grime

Wipe off any grime and dust with a rag or paper towel.

2. Call in Disinfectant

Spray the surface with your disinfecting solution of choice, and let it sit for 10 minutes. Wipe the disinfectant from the surface with a rag or paper towel.

3. Get a Streak-Free Finish

Use that favorite glass cleaner after disinfecting for streak- and spot-free glass. For a home-mixed glass cleaner, combine ¼ cup of vinegar in 3¾ cups of warm water in a spray bottle.

Whether applying store-bought or homemade cleaners, spray the glass cleaner lightly on a rag or paper towel and gently wipe the surface, using horizontal strokes on vertical surfaces to prevent dripping. Squeegee it dry. For extra sparkle, polish the surface when it's nearly dry with a piece of newspaper.

> **SANITIZING SURPRISE**
> **10 Minutes for You**
>
> Not everyone realizes that most disinfectants take about 10 minutes wet on the surface to truly go to work. Instead of looking at the process as a time suck, treat yourself to a simple act of self-care that you can do in 10 minutes while you wait. Read a chapter of a book. Sit down and drink a cup of *hot* tea for once. Or step outside and just breathe.

Resist the urge to clean any of your glass with abrasive cleaners, such as steel wool pads, as they can scratch surfaces.

METALS: MEET THE CHALLENGE

You don't need fancy household cleaners to tackle metal surfaces like aluminum, steel, copper, brass, and bronze. Plain old soap and water have the cleaning chops to bust away even the toughest dried-on or baked-on surface grime—with a little help in the elbow grease department from you. Use a sponge and apply some force, and you should be good to go.

Isopropyl alcohol is an excellent general disinfectant for metal surfaces. Just make sure its concentration is at least 70 percent. If the isopropyl alcohol is less than 70 percent concentration, it may not effectively eviscerate those nasty surface germs.

You can mix a 50-50 solution of water and rubbing alcohol to disinfect your hard-surface metals.

To use, spray or wipe the alcohol solution onto the metal surface and let sit for a minimum of 30 seconds to disinfect properly. Some cleaners and disinfectants, like bleach and vinegar-based solutions, can corrode the finish on certain metal surfaces. Avoid using these on any of your high-touch metal surfaces, such as chrome faucets, stainless-steel countertops, appliances, or cabinet handles or knobs.

Try these cleaning tips for all different types of metals.

Aluminum
Wash aluminum surfaces or objects with warm water and dish soap, using a sponge or rag to remove grease and some surface germs. Follow with your disinfecting alcohol solution.

Brass/Bronze
Soap and water work well here, too. Or break out a lime (or lemon) and salt. No, it's not margarita time (yet). Use these simple staples to provide both the acid and the abrasion needed to clean away surface dirt and grime. To use, rinse the surface so that it is wet enough for the salt to adhere. Sprinkle the salt liberally over the surface. Then grab the lemon or lime rind to scour the surface clean. Follow with your disinfecting alcohol solution.

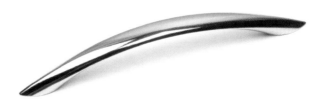

Chrome

Wash chrome surfaces with soap and water. Residue on faucets or handles can be removed with vinegar lightly dabbed on a microfiber cloth and briefly applied to the surface. Use a light touch here. Too much exposure to acids can cause corrosion on chrome surfaces. If you're too timid to try that, you can also use toothpaste. To use, squeeze a teaspoon-sized drop of toothpaste on a slightly damp microfiber cloth. Gently rub on the chrome surface. Wipe away toothpaste and buff dry. Follow with your disinfecting alcohol solution.

Natural Tarnish Remover

You might not think of ketchup as a cleaner, but its acidic nature makes it ideal for removing tarnish from brass, bronze, and copper. To use, find a bowl large enough to fit your item inside. Place it in the bowl and squeeze away until it is covered in layers of goopy ketchup. Use a sponge or microfiber cloth to gently clean the surface to remove tarnish. Remove your item from the ketchup and rinse thoroughly under running water in the sink. Towel dry.

Copper

Research shows that many viruses cannot survive on this surface for more than four hours thanks to its natural antimicrobial properties. Copper can be cleaned with soap and water and sanitized with isopropyl alcohol. To use, lightly dampen a microfiber cloth with the rubbing alcohol and give the surface a thorough wipe-down.

Stainless Steel

Approach stainless with a forceful surface scrubbing with soap and water. A 70 percent alcohol solution can both disinfect and act as a surface cleaner and degreaser. Avoid using vinegar on stainless steel, as the acidic properties can corrode the metal.

DON'T OVERLOOK
THESE METAL MENACES

Can Openers

Whether yours is an old-fashioned manual crank-turn model or a more modern electric gadget, the blade that cuts into the can inevitably touches the contents inside. Be sure to clean these appliances after each use with a damp cloth or sponge dipped in soapy water.

To clean an electric can opener: Unplug it and remove the cutting wheels (per the instruction manual). Soak those germy wheels in water with a few squirts of liquid dish soap. Remove any stubborn grime with a toothbrush. To clean the rest of the opener, apply a surface disinfectant following the product label's instructions.

To clean a manual can opener: Soak your manual opener in warm soapy water or, if dishwasher safe, send it through a cycle on the top rack. Dry thoroughly after cleaning to keep from rusting.

Doorknobs

While you'd probably like to think everyone in your house washes their hands faithfully every time they use the bathroom, make food, or come in from outside, chances are they don't. So every doorknob has a pretty good chance of harboring germs. It's not just the bathroom doorknob that's teeming with bacteria, viruses, and who knows what else. It's all the doorknobs and electronic keypads around the house, especially the front doorknob. No problem, a quick wipe-down with a disinfecting wipe will, well, wipe out the germy dilemma! One wipe per room, please. Efficient though these handy disinfectant cleaners may be, one can't disinfect a houseful of doorknobs.

PLASTICS: PUT GERMS IN THEIR PLACE

Our homes' ubiquitous plastic surfaces—children's and pets' toys, knobs, handles and touchpads, light switches, and kitchen appliances—are washable with a mild or neutral all-purpose detergent. A chlorine bleach solution is a safe and inexpensive disinfectant for most plastics, but test it first on an inconspicuous area before tackling the entire surface to make sure it doesn't cause any surface discoloration. Follow the manufacturer's instructions precisely when cleaning any electric appliance.

While plastic surfaces may seem indestructible, don't push the cleaning envelope here. Plastics can quickly be done in by harsh cleaners or strong acids that can cloud the surface. Mild cleaners are safest. Here's how to clean and disinfect plastic surfaces all around the house.

Kids' and Pets' Plastic Toys

Besides the visible dirt and grime, children's and pets' toys can harbor allergens and germs. How you clean and care for toys will depend on the surface material. Start by cleaning the surface with a sponge dipped in soapy water. Then most toys can withstand a light surface buffing daily with a disinfecting wipe. To tackle colorfast toys, you have a few options:

What's Feeding in That Pet Bowl?

If little Liam loves to play with the family pet, be aware that the germs collecting on Fido's toys and food and water bowls may pose a threat to family health. A recent study found bacteria—including *Salmonella*, *E. coli*, mold, mildew, yeast, and *Staphylococcus*—were also chowing down there.

Before the next kibble call, take a few minutes to sanitize the bowls and the area surrounding them.

Wash pet food and water bowls with hot soapy water or send them for a cycle in the dishwasher. If you're handwashing the bowls, mix 1/3 cup of bleach in 1 gallon of water in the sink or a bucket, and put the bowls in and let them soak for 10 minutes. Rinse thoroughly, then dry with a cloth or towel. Aim to sanitize pet bowls at least once a week.

- Disinfecting wipes

- A cloth dampened with a 3 percent hydrogen peroxide solution

- A bleach and water solution (follow the directions on the bleach label)

To be effective against germs, make sure the solution stays on the toy's surface for 10 full minutes, or as directed on the disinfecting product's label. Always mix or use a fresh bleach solution. Rinse the surface and dry thoroughly.

Solid plastic toys can also easily be cleaned in your dishwasher's top rack.

- Place larger toys securely between the tines in the rack.

- Put small toys into a mesh bag to keep them from moving around with the forceful water spray.

- Select the normal or sanitizing cycle and heated dry.

- After the cycle is complete, make sure to thoroughly air- or towel dry any toys that may come out of the dishwasher still wet.

Knobs, Handles, and Touchpads

How often are those knobs and handles in your kitchen, bedroom, and bathroom handled daily? The fridge door handles? The microwave touchpad? Are everyone's hands pristine each time? Probably not so much.

Contamination from foods and body soil leaves bacteria like *Salmonella*, *Listeria*, *E. coli*, yeast, and molds on these surfaces. These organisms can cause trouble of the tummy kind and are especially dire to young children and those with weakened immune systems.

After each meal or snack—or at least daily—use a disinfectant wipe or spray-on disinfectant cleaner on your kitchen cabinet hardware, appliance handles, and control panels to show germs who's boss. You can also use this easy-to-mix diluted bleach solution:

- For big families or hectic households: add ⅓ cup of bleach to 1 gallon of room-temperature water.

- Personal size: in a spray bottle, swirl together 4 teaspoons bleach and a quart of water.

Bleach solutions will be effective for disinfection for up to 24 hours.

Light Switches

Just about everyone in your home touches a light switch at some point each day. And the ones near your entrance doors are dirtier than, say, bedroom light switches, because we often arrive home with all sorts of germs on our hands. We won't even talk about what's lurking on the bathroom light switches.

Wipe all of your light switches and plates at least once a week with a disinfecting wipe or follow the instructions on a bottle of a spray disinfectant. Boost your disinfecting game to daily during periods of illness or flu season.

FLOORS: FEEL GOOD ABOUT CLEAN

I love walking into a room with clean and shiny floors. Who doesn't? But let's get real here. Our floors are a potluck of dirt, germs, and grime. Using the right cleaners for your floor's surface is critical in keeping these busy surfaces shining safely. But how do you know what you should use? There is a confusing array of floor-cleaning products on grocery store shelves. To determine the best cleaning solution for your floors, this guide can help.

Love That Linoleum

This retro cool flooring is made from organic materials (i.e., linseed oil, plus many additives including cork, pine resin, and minerals), and is antibacterial and non-allergenic. As a result,

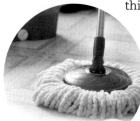

this is easy-peasy stuff. Damp-mop every few days or so. (Gentle reminder here: damp-mopping is not wet mopping.) Too much water exposure can make your linoleum floor brittle.

For really dirty jobs when a more in-depth cleaning is required, use a neutral pH cleaner, such as a few squirts of liquid dish soap in your mop bucket, and lightly go over the floor's surface.

CLEANING DON'TS: Hot water; strong alkaline cleaners, such as ammonia, bleach, or hydrogen peroxide; anything abrasive

Maintain a Vinyl Floor

Tiles or sheets of vinyl are soft to walk on and are available in many colors and patterns—some designed to look like granite, marble, wood, and other natural materials. All vinyl floors are coated with clear vinyl or urethane layers, making them relatively easy to keep clean and bright—as long as you keep daily dirt out of surface crevices, that is. Vacuum regularly to keep dust and grit from becoming ground in.

Clean regularly by damp-mopping with water only. When a deeper clean is needed, a cleaner with a surfactant will provide the muscle you need to get your floor clean. Or clean with ammonia and water, which also works well for a cork floor with a urethane finish.

CLEANING DON'TS: Anything soapy, such as mop-and-shine products; abrasive cleaners; paste wax

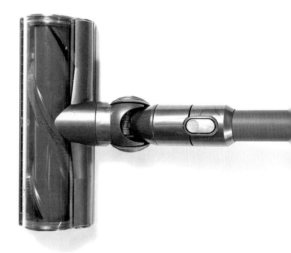

Handle Hardwood
Warm durable hardwood floors are easy to clean. Be sure to wipe up any liquid on the floor's surface promptly. The only other primary consideration is keeping grit and sand off the surface to keep scratches to a minimum.

Weekly, give the floor a thorough vacuuming. For a deeper clean, choose a wood floor cleaning product with a neutral pH. Wring the mop almost dry before mopping.

CLEANING DON'T: Standing water is the biggest threat to your gorgeous hardwood floor's longevity.

Keep Laminates Lovely

Laminates are hard materials consisting of two or more layers bonded together: a hard, thick base made of chipboard or similar material encased in a plastic laminate to get the look of hardwood without the cost and care.

Keep laminate floors clean by regularly vacuuming, dust-mopping, or wiping them with a damp (not wet) cloth. For tough dirt and grime, use a diluted vinegar solution. Buff away stubborn stains with undiluted acetone nail polish remover.

CLEANING DON'TS: Soap-based detergents (they'll make the floor slippery after cleaning) and abrasive cleaners or tools like steel wool (they can scratch the surface sheen)

Clean Natural Stone

Wipe or damp-mop natural stone floors daily to remove dust and tracked-in dirt. Even when sealed, these floors can be easily stained, especially by liquids. Make sure to wipe up spills as they happen throughout the day. For easier cleanups, hang the floor's damp mop in a nearby closet. Daily wipe-downs may seem cumbersome, but if you keep up with the cleaning, they'll continue looking lustrous for years.

CLEANING DON'TS: Dusting sprays or chemically treated mops or cloths; alkaline cleaners such as ammonia; strong soaps and detergents

Tame Terrazzo

This polished natural stone should be swept and damp-mopped with water and a few squirts of dishwashing liquid frequently to keep its surface sheen shiny. The cleaning bet here is to use the specialty products recommended by the manufacturer.

Treat Tiles Right

Regularly vacuum and damp-mop to remove dirt, dust, and sand to prevent ground-in grunge from scratching the shiny surface. For a deeper clean, use a neutral pH cleaner to keep the shiny finish intact.

CLEANING DON'TS: Standing moisture can cause damage; mop up any spills as soon as possible.

WALLS: CHASE HIDING GERMS

Your walls may not look like they need a good bath. After all, dirt and airborne germs fall to the floor, don't they? Much of them do, but just enough clings to vertical surfaces to warrant a monthly bath, especially for those walls around and behind the toilet.

A Super-Flusher Event

Flushing spreads germs throughout the air, which can be detected for close to 90 minutes. Being diligent and closing the lid helps, but many people (especially kids) don't remember to do it. For that reason, it's best not to keep toothbrushes, rinse cups, contact lens cases, or other toiletries within six feet of your toilet. Call it social distancing from germs.

Around the Toilet

To sanitize the walls around and behind the toilet, you'll need a sponge, two buckets (one for your soapy water solution, the other for rinsing the cleaning sponge), dishwashing liquid, and a microfiber cloth for drying.

1. SOAP UP A SPONGE

Dip your sponge in the bucket of soapy water, wring it slightly (so it isn't dripping), and start sponging the walls clean, working your way around from top to bottom.

2. RINSE THE SPONGE

Dunk into your fresh-water bucket as needed between wipes. Don't forget to wring the sponge out a bit to avoid drips. Then end with one final pass with fresh water to rinse the solution from your walls.

3. DRY THOROUGHLY

The microfiber cloth makes this easy work. It's important to chase away any last bits of moisture to avoid a setting that invites bacteria.

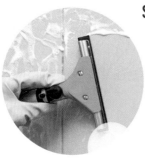

Shower Walls

Shower walls and tub floors are germy hot spots despite being inundated regularly with soap and water. The average bathtub is even dirtier than a trash can. That's because the dead skin cells, skin oils, stray hairs, and all the other stuff we're washing off our bodies get mingled with the fats in soap and shampoo. Then, voilà—biohazard! Although that hairy gunk could be swimming in germs, cleanup will not require protective gear other than a pair of cleaning gloves.

To keep germs in check and your tub clean, rinse it out after each bath to remove soil or soap residue. If it's only mildly dirty, you can just use soap and water with a microfiber cloth.

For shower walls and surrounds, keep a squeegee in the shower for quick post-shower wipe-downs. This is the best time to clean, as the steam from your shower will have loosened up any dried-on soap scum. A few passes with the squeegee, and down the drain it goes.

At least once a month, use a disinfectant on all tubs and surrounding areas to kill lingering germs.

TOILETS: TACKLE WITH EASE

Flush with reasons not to tackle the requisite weekly toilet tune-up? Have a seat and relax. If you haven't tackled a toilet in a while, you'll find it isn't quite so tedious these days, thanks to a new generation of disinfecting cleaners that do much of the scrubbing for you. I'm not saying it's a breeze (or a breath of fresh air), but it's not the monster of a chore it once was, with all that heavy scrubbing.

First, you'll want to properly suit up in protective gloves of rubber or latex. Then . . .

1. Hit the Toilet Bowl

Grab your disinfecting toilet bowl cleaner. It's a hard worker that does two jobs—cleans and disinfects. Squeeze or spray it around the bowl's interior. The bowl cleaner needs 10 minutes to do its dirty work, which is good because you have a few more surfaces to hit here.

2. Turn to the Seat

While the disinfectant is doing its job in the bowl, clean the seat and lid (both sides) and the rest of the toilet exterior, including around the hinges and the base. Spray on a nonabrasive disinfectant. This one needs 10 minutes, too.

> **CLEAN CHOICES**
> **Paper Towels versus Cloths**
>
> In a lot of cleaning endeavors, cleaning cloths or rags work just fine, as long as you launder properly soon after use. But the bathroom is one place where you might feel better using paper towels strategically and tossing them and the nasties they've removed immediately in the trash.

3. Return to the Bowl

Going back to bowl duty, grab a long-handled toilet bowl brush, open the lid, and swish the bowl cleaner around inside and as far into the trap as you can. Flush to rinse clean.

4. Seconds for the Seat

Time for another pass at the seat. Using paper towels, wipe the toilet seat clean. Then do the same to the bowl's exterior. Be sure to hit the bumpers and hinge areas in the back.

5. Go the Extra Mile

For weekly maintenance, you can pour a cup of baking soda in the bowl to keep it fresh.

To fight tough toilet stains, pour in about a half-gallon of white distilled vinegar. Let it soak overnight before flushing.

Now that wasn't too hard—doing battle with germs on your home's hard surfaces—was it? I didn't think so. Great! Let's take a walk on the softer side of cleaning porous surfaces in Chapter 4.

DON'T FORGET THE BIN

No matter how meticulous you are about lining the trash can with bags, some icky stuff inevitably seems to work its way to the bottom and sides of the can over time. To keep grime and germs from building up inside, make cleaning the bin a part of your weekly cleaning routine.

1. Don your handy cleaning gloves.

2. After you've removed the trash bag but before placing a new one inside, place the can in the shower or take it outside to clean.

3. Rinse the can interior thoroughly with warm soapy water.

4. Use a scrubber sponge or brush to loosen and remove any stubborn gunk that has adhered to the can's base or sides.

5. Rinse and allow the can to dry. If possible, air-dry it in the sun to disinfect naturally.

Spraying the interior with a disinfectant is still recommended.

THE SOFTER SIDE

How to Clean & Disinfect Porous Surfaces

THE SOFT SURFACES IN OUR HOMES—the carpet that feels so cozy under our feet, that sofa we can't wait to curl up on after a long day at work—help make our house feel like a home. But how do they fit into our cleaning scene?

For some time now, we have been diligently cleaning and disinfecting our homes' surfaces to keep germs in check and our families healthy. Going about your daily disinfecting routine, carefully sidestepping the sofa and living room chairs on your way to the kitchen countertops, you might have wondered: Will my disinfectant work on upholstery?

Soft porous surfaces like upholstered furniture, carpeting, and plush toys are a tough lot to clean. Take your comfy couch, for instance. While the soft porous fabric makes it dreamy to lounge on, it also makes it a veritable nightmare to disinfect, as the interwoven fibers provide plenty of places for pathogens to hide. Compare that to hard nonporous surfaces like the kitchen counters, where there is nowhere for microorganisms to run and hide. So, what's a clean freak to do with all of the soft spots around the house?

The Environmental Protection Agency (EPA), the regulating body for all things disinfectant, says no product (so far) can claim to completely disinfect couches, carpeting, or other soft surfaces. But as the role that soft surfaces play in germ transmission is becoming more evident, the EPA has created a new category of disinfectants with a soft-surface *sanitizing* claim. These products kill 99.9 percent of vegetative bacteria, like *Bordetella* and *Lepto-spira*, on soft surfaces. The catch: disinfectants kill viruses and fungi, too. So, while these products offer a start into new sanitizing efforts, they are not without their germ holes where risk can enter.

All is not lost, however. There is hope and a less-germy future ahead for your carpets and upholstery. While there's no guarantee one of these new sanitizers will rid the soft surfaces in your home of all pathogens, the cleaning process itself will go a long way in keeping germ risk under control. This chapter is filled with ways to safely clean soft surfaces in and around your home—from carpets, rugs, and upholstery to purses, backpacks, and plush toys.

CARPETS AND RUGS: CLEAN UNDER YOUR FEET

Our home's carpets and rugs see a lot of action daily. We and our pets track in contaminants on our shoes, in addition to the bodily fluids that collect from sneezes and coughs throughout the day. As a result, our carpets and rugs are often teeming with viruses, bacteria, and fungi waiting for us to pad around barefoot at bedtime so they can hitch a ride.

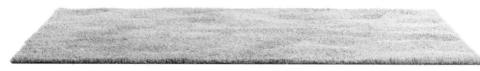

While it is impossible to kill all the microorganisms on (or disinfect) soft nonwashable surfaces like carpets and upholstery, you can sanitize most of these surfaces, significantly reducing bacteria levels and contamination. Here's how to keep the carpet in your home clean.

Become a Fan of Doormats

Place doormats at every entrance to your home. You might also want to consider instituting a "no shoes inside" policy. As recent studies have revealed, our shoes' soles can harbor all sorts of pathogens, including COVID-19 and other viruses. Shoes that have been outside can track in germs and grime from asphalt, pet droppings, dirt, and worse.

Safe Soft Sanitizing

When shampooing carpets or upholstery using a new or borrowed cleaning machine, test it out first on an inconspicuous area of your carpet or sofa to ensure the treatment won't discolor the sofa's fabric or the carpet fibers.

Suck It Up

Vacuum carpet and upholstery at least twice a week, more frequently in heavily trafficked areas and during cold and flu season. (Sorry!) The next time you pull out the machine, keep in mind that effectively sucking up and removing the dirt and germs hidden in carpet and upholstery fibers requires about 20 seconds of going back and forth over each area. Change bags often, and keep the vacuum's beater bar and brushes clean.

Don't Skip Shampoos

Shampoo or have your carpets professionally cleaned at least twice a year; seasonally is better. If someone in your home is ill with an infectious disease, or if you have a dust-allergy sufferer in residence, more frequent deep cleaning is recommended.

You can save time when shampooing by shifting furniture a few inches instead of hauling every stick of furniture you own into the far corners of the room like your mom probably did. Place protective coasters (or wax paper squares) beneath furniture legs to protect your carpet and keep your furniture dry while the carpet is drying. After shampooing, throw open the windows to allow fresh air to circulate. This can shave hours off your carpet's drying time, which can take up to 48 hours without this assistance.

If all this still sounds like a bit too much work, you do have options here. Call that carpet cleaning company down the street and take the day off.

Know When to Wash

Unlike wall-to-wall carpets, some small area rugs can be cleaned and disinfected in the washing machine. Before sending a rug for a spin in the washer, however, take it and shake it—outside, that is. Or beat it with a broom to dislodge surface dirt and debris.

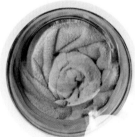

A front-loading washer or a top-load model without a center agitator can accommodate a larger area rug better than a standard top-load washer. You might want to consider heading to a laundromat that has larger washers. Choose the hottest water recommended on the rug's care label. Add a laundry detergent containing enzymes and a laundry disinfectant (such as a name-brand laundry sanitizer, pine oil, or chlorine bleach) following product directions. If the carpet does not have a rubber backing, tumble dry on high heat. If the rug cannot withstand the heat, allow it to air-dry.

UPHOLSTERY:
SANITIZING YOUR SOFA AND MORE

Fabrics that have absorbed a season's worth (or longer) of dirt, body oil, and germs need a bath to get them ready for another season of entertaining—and for that close inspection from visiting friends and family.

Before you begin, locate the manufacturer's care tag on the sofa cushions or chair to see its recommended method of overall cleaning. Much like clothes care labels with symbols that communicate washing and drying instructions, upholstery has its own cleaning code, one that is often hard to decipher. (If your upholstered furniture doesn't have a code, test a cleaner on a hidden spot first.)

Here's how to decipher what you're likely to see on your upholstery care labels:

O = Clean with cold water because the upholstery is made from organic materials.

S = Clean with a mild water-free dry-cleaning solvent. Use just a little solvent, and make sure you have plenty of ventilation. Do not use water or water-based products on this item.

W = Clean with a water-based product, such as a little foam from a mild detergent or nonsolvent upholstery shampoo. Use as little foam and water as possible to do the job; you don't want to get the upholstery too wet. Moisture encourages mold, mildew, and bacteria to take up residence.

WS = You can use a dry-cleaning solvent, the foam of a mild detergent, or upholstery shampoo.

X = Don't clean it yourself. You can, however, vacuum or brush off surface grime. Hire a professional when a deeper cleaning is required.

When you're ready to clean upholstered furniture, you can follow four basic steps.

1. Start with a Vacuum
Vacuum the surface, cushions, the body below the cushions (where crumbs, quarters, and remote controls hide), and behind and under the furniture piece. Then brush with an upholstery brush to dislodge surface dirt and dust, following the vacuum path so you don't miss any area. Vacuum the dislodged dirt.

2. Get on a Roll
Go over the main body and cushions with a lint roller, following the path of the vacuum and brush. This will bring out stubborn pet hair and resistant dust.

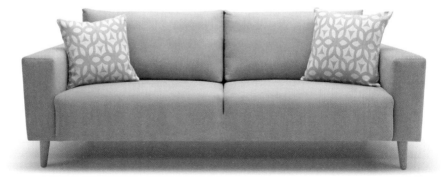

3. Clean with Foam

This step is for water-tolerant upholstery only—do not use if your upholstery is coded S or X.

Whip equal parts dishwashing liquid and water. Apply the resulting foam to the upholstery. Gently work the foam into the upholstery with your fingertips so as not to strain the fabric. Let it sit for 5 minutes.

4. Blot-Rinse (Don't Saturate)

Again, this step is for water-tolerant uphol-stery only—do not use if your upholstery is coded S or X.

Remove the soapy foam from the cleaned areas using a sponge dampened with water. This will be easier if you have a bucket of clean water handy. Blot dry with a microfiber or cotton cloth, soaking up as much moisture as you can. Let air-dry completely before the family takes a seat.

> **CLEAN CHOICES**
> **Store-Bought Product versus Your Pantry**
>
> Carpet and upholstery freshening powders exist, but it's so easy to make your own natural solution. If you really want to impress fellow clean freaks, quickly remove any lingering sofa odors with baking soda. Using a cheese shaker, sprinkle a thin layer of baking soda over carpets or upholstered surfaces. Let sit for 15 minutes or overnight, then vacuum clean. Aren't you the thorough one!

PURSES AND BAGS: KICK OUT GERMS

We are all guilty of putting our handbags down in some rather unsavory places from time to time. Sometimes when we're in small spaces (like bathroom stalls), we just put it wherever it's most convenient. All the places we leave it—on car floorboards, movie theater and restaurant floors, dirty counters—explain those icky travelers on the outside.

The purse's exterior isn't the only part that's prone to host potential nasties—the inside attracts a lot of dirt, too. Does stuffing your purse to the brim with random items and only cleaning it once in a blue moon ring a bell, anyone? As a result, there's more than crumpled receipts and spare change lurking inside. When

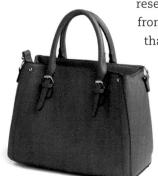

researchers carried out detailed tests on 145 handbags from 80 women and 65 men, results showed that more than 90 percent of the bags had bacteria contamination. Women were the worst offenders: bacteria growth was higher on women's purses than on men's bags.

A big part of the problem is that we often forget to clean our handbags—or worse yet, we don't think about it at all. That bag study found that less than 3 percent of the women cleaned their purses monthly. The danger: some nasty bacteria—*Staphylococcus*, *Micrococcus*, *Bacillus*, and *Enterococcus*—can colonize on handbags and can lead to staph infections, septic shock, meningitis, ear infections, urinary tract infections (UTIs), and more.

The solution is simple: buck the curve and start cleaning your purse. Weekly would be an admirable goal, but monthly is respectable. Your cleaning options:

WASH IT. Some handbags are machine washable. If you carry one of them, toss it in the next time you're running a load.

WIPE IT. Synthetic bags are a cinch to clean. Dump out the gunk, vacuum inside, and run an antibacterial wipe or two along the entire outer surface.

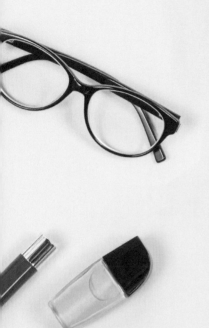

MINIMIZE GERMY PURSE RISK

Don't stress—the takeaway here isn't that you should obsessively sterilize your handbag. Just because bacteria can cause you to get sick doesn't mean they will. Here's how to protect yourself and your purse in simple ways.

CHOOSE SAFE HOMES. Designate a hook or shelf near the entry door to hang or stash your purse on. That way, you'll avoid picking up—or dropping off—bacteria via the germ-laden kitchen counter. Don't toss it on your bed, either, where it could spread germs throughout your bedroom.

WATCH WHAT GOES INSIDE. If you need to bring your workout shoes or lunch with you on the way out the door, bag them in protective plastic before you put them inside. Food and shoes can provide a fertile growing ground for bacteria. Your purse might just smell better, too.

KEEP UP WITH THE HAND HYGIENE. Regularly wash your hands or use that hand sanitizer in your purse, and you'll sleep better at night knowing you've done everything within your power to stay healthy.

And if you prefer leather, know that your purse material of choice does safeguard you from excess bacteria buildup better than other options. (Yay!) The only downside to leather (other than the price) is that you can't safely use antibacterial cleaning solvents on them without stripping its finish or color. What you can do is wipe down its fabric lining with hot soapy water and use a leather conditioner to keep it pretty on the outside, too.

MAKEUP APPLICATORS: CLEAN BRUSHES AND SPONGES

Your hands likely touch your face the most, but applicators used to apply makeup also have plenty of opportunity to transfer germs. Cleaning your brushes and sponges not only removes dirt and bacteria, it helps them stand up to their important tasks of making you look beautiful and may help them last longer (good news for your budget). To prevent the spread of germs, wash your hands well before applying makeup, and clean your applicators weekly.

Better Brushes

How you clean makeup brushes depends on what they're made of. Natural brushes hold on to bacteria tighter yet need gentler care. For these, it may be best to turn to store-bought cleaners specially designed for your brushes and to follow product label directions. You can find types that enable you to dip your brushes in a solution, ones that you shampoo them in and then rinse, and still others to spritz on the brushes and then wipe off.

Synthetic brushes are less prone to accumulating bacteria and easier to clean and dry quickly. One good DIY disinfectant: add a teaspoon of hydrogen peroxide and a few drops of baby shampoo to a bowl of warm water. Allow your brushes to soak in the

76

solution for about 10 minutes, then swish and remove. Rinse with cold water.

Make sure to allow your brushes to air-dry completely before putting them back into the makeup application rotation. Moisture encourages bacteria.

For daily sanitizing of both natural and synthetic brushes, spray a tissue with alcohol and wipe the brush on the tissue.

Makeup Blending Sponges

These workhorse sponges enable you to apply just a bit of foundation or concealer to cover, well, everything you want to cover. But after a week, they can hide a lot of product and bacteria. To bring a blender back to the clean side, squeeze it under running water until it is completely soaked. Apply a squirt of dishwashing liquid or baby shampoo directly on the sponge, then massage it in as you press it gently with your hands. Enjoy the satisfaction of all that makeup mess releasing, then rinse and wring until the water runs clear. Allow to air-dry completely.

Another clever way to approach that blender: Treat it like a kitchen sponge and zap it. Just like your microwave can kill germs on that dish sponge, it can help sanitize your beauty sponge as well. This sponge will need a bit more moisture to keep it safe as it's sanitized. Fill a microwave-safe cup with water, then add a few squirts of dish soap or baby shampoo. Put the beauty sponge in the cup, dipping it a few times in the solution to get it nice and wet. Microwave for 1 minute, let it cool 30 seconds before removing, then allow it to cool fully before lifting out the sponge and rinsing under running water. Wring out and allow to air-dry.

KID STUFF:
SANITIZE BACKPACKS, TOYS & MORE

Kids have a lot of soft stuff—from book bags to plush toys—and their germy stuff needs cleaning and sanitizing, too. Of course it does—it belongs to kids! No matter how many times you remind them about germs, virus- and bacteria-fighting are not at the top of their priority list. But there are simple ways you can stop the germs they introduce (cover that sneeze!) and bring in—from childcare, school, friends' houses, sports practices, and the dirt pile they discovered in the backyard—from spreading all through your home.

Clean Busy Backpacks

Every day, several times a day, those backpacks get tossed on the floor or filled with dirty items. Now imagine what else has touched those floors. The straps harbor the bacteria from everything your child's hands have touched throughout the day. When they toss that backpack on the kitchen counter or table, all those germs and bacteria come along.

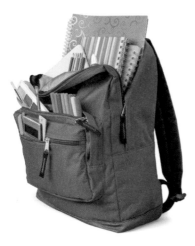

To clean backpacks, first empty the interior of lunch remnants, last month's homework, and other detritus. Then form a thorough cleaning plan. Many backpacks and book bags are washable and come with laundering instructions. If the backpack or book bag can be washed, follow label instructions (if still legible), or wash it weekly in the warmest water safe for the fabric. If not washable, take a disinfecting wipe to the interior and exterior weekly.

Target Plush Toys

Simply constructed plush toys—without built-in battery packs, noisemakers, or other metal parts—are generally machine washable. Plush toys can go for a whirl in the dryer, too. Always check any care labels for guidance first.

To wash plush playtime favorites, make sure all teddy's decorations and buttons are securely attached and repair any rips or holes before sending him for a spin. Place plush toys inside a zip-close mesh laundry bag to protect them. Select the machine's sanitizing cycle, if it has one, or warm water.

Dry on high heat until fully dry. Another option: Break out the hair dryer. Start with a low heat setting, and when nearly dry, switch to medium heat and fluff out his fur.

Don't Forget Pet Toys

If Fido has his favorite soft toys, give them a bath, too. Wash colorfast soft pet toys monthly, or on an as-needed basis, in hot water with laundry detergent containing enzymes and a laundry sanitizer (such as a brand-name product, pine oil, or chlorine bleach), following product directions.

Chase Germs Off Car Seats

Kids' car seats, according to one study, are home to more germs than your toilet! Nasties riding along with your child include norovirus, *E. coli*, *Salmonella*, and cold and flu germs. To clean your child's car seat:

- First, read the manufacturer's instruction guide for the specific do's and don'ts for your seat model.

- Wipe away dried-on dirt, food, and the like from the surface with a damp cloth.

- Wipe the harness straps clean with a disinfecting wipe or remove them and spot clean with soapy water.

- Take off the cloth cover and wash it in cool water on your machine's delicate cycle. Let the cover air-dry. Machine drying is generally not recommended; it could shrink.

- Take out the seat buckle and wipe with a disinfectant wipe; allow to air-dry. After you reinstall the buckle, give it a few pulls to make sure it fastens correctly.

Don't use bleach to clean your child's car seat. Bleach could strip away the protective flame retardant.

Sanitize Sports Equipment

Our sporty kids require seemingly endless gear to pursue their activity of choice. While parents love the protection these accessories provide our children, the smelly germy messes they often become after months of use . . . not so much. Everything gets covered in sweat, stored on locker room floors, and before long, they're swimming in germs that could make them sick.

The problems don't end when they hit the showers. Shower room floors are often a breeding ground for mold and fungi if they aren't cleaned properly. Fungi and viruses here are the types that can cause plantar warts, staph infections, athlete's foot, colds and flu, and ringworm.

Handy Helper

No matter how much you scrub all the kid equipment, practicing good hand hygiene—especially with babies in residence—is still probably the most powerful way to prevent the spread of germs and to keep everyone in the family healthy, especially during cold and flu seasons.

To keep kids healthy while they're actively out and about:

- Invest in a pair of protective shower shoes, such as slip-resistant flip-flops or sandals, for your swimmer or team player, so they can avoid walking barefoot in shared shower and locker room areas.

- Make sure her gym bag is always stocked with a fresh post-workout change of clothes.

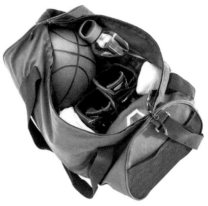

- To clean sports helmets and pads at home, use non-chemical cleaning solutions like white vinegar to destroy odors and surface bacteria. You can also use sanitizing cleaning wipes.

- Clothes, socks, and shoe pads can be laundered with a sanitizer and dried.

- When the gym bag comes home, remind your child to immediately remove that sweaty uniform or wet swimsuit for washing. And, while you're at it, set the gym bag in a well-ventilated place to enable it to air out and air-dry. Allowing bags to dry out between uses helps prevent the growth of mold and bacteria inside.

DON'T FORGET YOUR CLEANING SUPPLIES

I can hear it now: "You mean I have to clean *cleaning* supplies?" Yes, you need to clean cleaning supplies, too—if you want to win the war against household dirt, grime, and germs in your home and keep your family healthy, that is. A filthy mop will only redeposit dirt or just move it around on your floor each time you use it. Grimy rags will leave surface streaks.

Here's how to clean your all-important cleaning tools—brooms, dusters, mop heads, toilet brushes, sponges, and cotton and microfiber cleaning cloths—so you make the most of your precious cleaning time.

Freshen Brooms

A broom and dustpan might seem like a quaint idea from back in the day, but for little cleanups around the house, a broom is just the thing. Whether yours is microfiber or extruded plastic, the broom's bristles need to be cleaned regularly to remove trapped dirt and dust.

To deep clean, mix a bucket of hot water and three to four quick squirts of dishwashing liquid. Swirl the broom and dustpan through the solution to clean. Rinse thoroughly. To dry, store the broom with the bristles down and place a bucket beneath it to capture the drips. When dry, store the broom with the bristles up to maintain a crisp edge.

De-Dust Dusters

After using, take your duster outside and give it a good shaking for a minute or so. It helps to tap the handle firmly to loosen dust.

To deep clean, swirl the duster through a bucket of warm water and several squirts of dishwashing liquid for a minute or two, just as you did with the broom. Rinse thoroughly, and squeeze excess water out. Drip dry, or place the duster in a jar with the fluffy side up. For extra fluffing, use a blow dryer on the lowest setting to dry it for 2 minutes.

Sock It to Dust

Save orphaned or stretched-out socks for a second life as a hands-on dust cloth. Don them like gloves, spray them with water or polish, and off you go! When one side gets dusty, just flip the sock and continue using the other side. Cleanup is a cinch, too: toss the sock in the washing machine with hot water and chlorine bleach, following label instructions.

Clean Mop Heads

Whether made of cotton, sponge, or microfiber fabric, mop heads should be cleaned thoroughly after each use to remove dirt and debris from the fibers. This is because once the fibers are saturated with soil, your mop head cannot efficiently gather or mop up additional dirt, dust, or debris, leaving filthy streaks on your floors.

Removable cotton and microfiber mop heads can be sent for a spin in the washer in hot water with a heavy-duty laundry detergent to remove embedded grease and soil. Add ½ cup of chlorine bleach to the wash to disinfect. Hang or lay flat to air-dry. Wait until the fibers are completely dry to return it to the cleaning cache.

For non-removable fabric mop heads, soak for 15 minutes in hot water and detergent or pine oil cleaner in a bucket or sink. Then move the head around to loosen the soil. Rinse thoroughly and allow to air-dry. If the mop head smells funky, add ⅓ cup of chlorine bleach per gallon of rinse water to disinfect the fibers.

After using your sponge mop, rinse it thoroughly under hot, running water. To disinfect, submerge the mop in a solution of ⅓ cup of chlorine bleach per gallon of water for 10 minutes. Wearing gloves to protect your hands, agitate to loosen dirt and soil. Rinse the mop thoroughly, then press and squeeze out excess water. Allow to air-dry.

Buckets Need Baths, Too

After use, always rinse a bucket with hot water to flush away whatever grime you just removed. To disinfect, first fill the bucket with water. Then, following label directions, add chlorine bleach, pine oil, or phenolic disinfectant (such as Lysol). Let the mixture sit for 10 minutes. Donning a pair of gloves to protect your hands, clean inside and outside surfaces of the bucket with a scrub brush. Don't forget the handle!

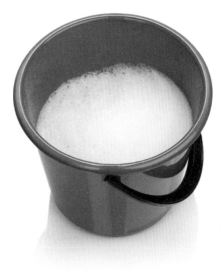

Tackle the Toilet Brush

There's actually a relatively painless way to complete this often unpleasant chore. Remove the brush from its caddy (if it has one) and soak it in a diluted bleach solution. My favorite shortcut is adding 1 cup of bleach to a toilet bowl full of clean water, then letting the brush soak inside for an hour or so. When time is up, I flush the toilet to rinse the bowl and brush. Let the brush drip dry into the toilet bowl, sandwiched under the toilet seat. Let the brush dry completely before putting it back in the toilet brush holder.

Speaking of the toilet brush holder . . . you'll want to clean it, too. Disinfecting one without the other kind of defeats the purpose. While the toilet brush is soaking, wipe or spray a disinfectant on the holder's interior and exterior. Allow it to sit for the amount of time suggested on the product's label, then wipe clean with paper towels.

Sanitize Your Sponge

Your handy cleaning sponge is hands down one of the dirtiest things in your house. Go figure—it's wet, absorbent, and you rub dirt and food on it day in and day out.

By definition, sponges, whether natural or humanmade, are a porous material. While those pores are what makes them so great for absorbing spills, they are also quite adept at holding on to moisture and bacteria, creating the perfect growing ground for illness-causing germs.

To clean and disinfect your sponge, fill a bucket or sink with water and ⅓ cup of bleach per gallon of water. Toss in the sponge for a 5-minute soak. Then rinse, squeeze out excess water, and air-dry in a well-ventilated area. In testing, the bleach solution killed 99.9 percent of bacteria strains from sponges.

Microwaving your sponge is another effective method of sponge disinfection. It was equally effective, zapping 99.9 percent of sponge germs in 2 quick minutes. To use this method, make sure your sponge is moist or place your sponge in water (¼ cup for scrub sponges and ½ cup for cellulose sponges), then zap on high for 2 minutes. You may want to let it chill in the microwave for a few minutes before retrieving; it emerges very hot. To guard against the risk of fire, only zap sponges that are without metallic content.

Sponges should be cleaned weekly. But no matter how diligent you are about cleaning, they won't last forever. If the sponge has a funky odor after cleaning, replace it. That odor is a sign of excessive bacterial growth. And even if it doesn't smell, its life span in your kitchen should be two weeks, max. Out with the old, and in with the new!

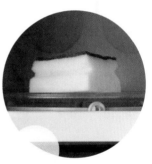

Launder Cleaning Cloths

Both cotton and microfiber types come in handy on chore day. Microfiber cleaning cloths are a polyester and nylon cloth blend offered in various textures and weaves designed to clean different surfaces, including mirrors, windows, and stainless steel. I use microfiber cleaning cloths because they don't leave lint or surface streaks behind after use. Because they are washable, they're an economical choice. Cotton cloths are the workhorses of cleaning cloths, just the thing for heavy-duty cleaning jobs around the home that involve oily or strong cleaners. Another plus: they're more sanitary than sponges.

Cotton cloths can be machine washed in hot water with laundry detergent and chlorine bleach (following label instructions) to remove soil and disinfect. If a cloth is saturated with grease or cleaning products, presoak it in hot water and a degreaser before washing. And, keep it out of the dryer. Even after washing, oil-soaked cotton cloths are combustible. Simply allow to air-dry instead.

You can also machine wash and dry microfiber cloths to get them ready for their next round of cleaning action. Just don't use a fabric softener in the wash water or dryer sheet in the dryer, as fabric softener diminishes the dust-attracting qualities of the fibers.

Now that your cleaning supplies are ready for sanitizing action, let's examine your electronics in Chapter 5. Electronics can be areas we tend to ignore because we're unsure how to safely clean all those screens and speakers. But no more, with step-by-step strategies coming up!

REFRESH SHOWER CURTAINS

Don't forget to clean hardworking shower curtains. Each week or so, send washable shower curtains and liners for a spin in the washing machine. Use warm water and add bleach to the wash water to loosen and remove mildew, mold, and soap scum. Before rehanging, give the curtain a good soak in a salt-water solution to prevent mildew. The easiest way to do this: Put the curtain in your clean bathtub and run enough water to fully submerge the curtain. As the water runs, add 1 cup of salt. Let the curtain sit in the soak anywhere from 10 minutes to a few hours, depending on the time you can afford. Then drain, rehang, and allow to dry in place.

Clean polyester and plastic shower curtains and liners where they hang using a laundry prewash spray or detergent solution (1 teaspoon of laundry detergent per 1 cup of water). Simply spray the solution all along the top of the curtain so it drips down and covers the entire curtain. Let it sit for a few minutes and go to work. Then rinse clean and allow to air-dry.

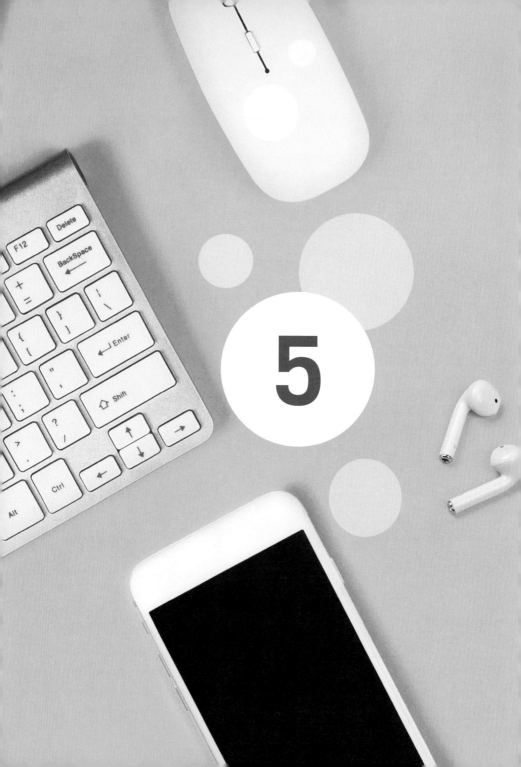

5

FOCUS ON ELECTRONICS

How to Sanitize Cell Phones, Computers, Remotes & More

WE'RE SPENDING MORE TIME ON OUR CELL PHONES, computers, and other personal electronics than ever—items that even before the pandemic were notorious for their germy surfaces. Still, for most of us, the first thing we thought about when someone asked, "Have you ever cleaned up your cell phone?" was how to remove junk files and the plethora of bad photos to free up storage space.

What a difference a pandemic makes! The first thing that comes to mind now about cleaning a cell phone is purely physical—removing the legion of potential illness-causing microbes and bacteria teeming on its surface. It's something few of us did pre-pandemic, probably because we just weren't sure how.

After all, we all know our electronic devices require special care when it comes to cleaning. With electronics, even a stray drop of water can sound the death knell. But you don't need to stress—let the solutions in this chapter help you safely sanitize your cell phone, computers, and remotes, and give all your gadgets a good general cleaning. Channel your inner germaphobe—you've got this!

CELL PHONES & MORE: SCREEN GERMS

It's enough to make a germaphobe gag: scientists at the University of Arizona found cell phones have on average ten times more bacteria than a toilet seat. It's easy enough to understand why—we're practically joined at the hip (or ear or arm) with our cell phones. Our smartphones keep us running. They have become the remote control to our lives—from staying in touch with family and friends to setting reminders and even waking up in the morning. Where we go, they go, too. And, let's be honest here, we occasionally hang out at some rather unsavory places (think public restrooms). As a result, our cell phones tend to get pretty gross.

Clean Hands, Clean Devices

When possible, make sure you wash your hands after texting and before you eat. And again, after eating and before texting. The first thing you should do when cleaning electronics is make sure your hands are clean. You know the drill: wash your hands with soap and water for a minimum of 20 seconds. Clean hands will keep you from transferring additional germs to the surface you're trying to clean.

Our own hands are the biggest culprit when it comes to the filth that gets on our phones. According to a recent study, we check our phones every 12 minutes—or 80 times a day. We provide ample opportunities for pathogens, including *Streptococcus*, MRSA, and *E. coli*, to move from our fingers to our phones. Once settled in, these microscopic menaces can live for hours on a warm surface like your phone or tablet. It's time to send those bad boys packing—stat!

A lightly dampened cloth is often enough to get rid of surface smears and fingerprints on your cell phone and other touchscreens. To remove all the microscopic menaces, however, requires a two-step approach: cleaning and disinfecting. Yes, cleaning and disinfecting are separate processes. Cleaning physically removes surface dust, dirt, and smudges, and many, but not all, germs. Disinfecting kills those left behind.

Follow these steps to safely get your cell phone, tablet, and other touchscreen devices grime-free using an easy-to-make, inexpensive electronics cleaning and sanitizing spray.

1. Power Off, Wipe Off

Always start by powering off your device. Not only is it easier to see dirt and smudges when the screen is off, but it is safer, too. Also, remove the device's case. It's better to clean and disinfect them separately, so you don't miss any crevices that germs are calling home.

Thoroughly yet gently wipe the screen and surfaces with a soft, dry (or *very lightly* water-dampened) lint-free cloth or microfiber cloth to remove smudges, dust, and debris. Avoid scrubbing vigorously, as this might cause damage. Be sure to clean both the front and back of the device and the case.

2. Clear the Crevices

Now, we're getting down to the real dirty business. First, use a toothbrush to remove dust and other debris in the crevices around your phone or tablet's screen.

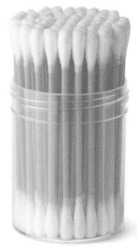

To remove dirt in speaker holes and the cord connection area, use one of your vacuum cleaner's small attachments to suck away the offending debris. (Don't use compressed air because you could inadvertently drive the dirt farther into the device holes.)

THE LATEST ON SAFE SCREEN CLEANING

If you haven't been cleaning touchscreens as much as you should, it could be because the methods sometimes seem to be a moving target. Here's what you need to know about what's recently been determined safe to use and what is still not safe to use.

PUT AWAY THE WINDEX

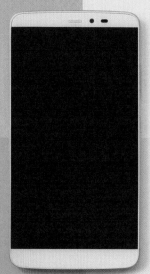

Your first instinct upon encountering a smudged screen of any kind might be to grab the glass cleaner and go to town. Resist that urge at all costs. Any touch-sensitive screens have an oleophobic coating to resist smudging and fingerprints. Chemicals, like ammonia, in most glass cleaners are adept at not only removing surface grease and grime on glass but eradicating that protective surface coating on your electronic devices.

WIPES ARE OKAY

For anyone with an iPhone, you'll be interested to know that early into the pandemic, in March 2020, Apple updated its cleaning guidelines to encourage the use of isopropyl alcohol to kill bacteria, viruses, and other pathogenic microbes on its products. You may recall that before the update rubbing alcohol was a big no-no.

Big companies like Apple changed their tune on disinfecting screens during the pandemic. While Apple used to advise against using bleach-based cleaners and similar agents on its products' screens, it's now urging customers to use them to be safer.

The revised cleaning guidelines now endorse using "a 70 percent isopropyl alcohol wipe or Clorox Disinfecting Wipes" to gently wipe the hard, nonporous electronic surfaces, such as the display and keyboard and other exterior surfaces. Further recommendations, according to Apple: "Don't use bleach. Avoid getting moisture in any opening, don't spray cleaners directly on the surface, and don't submerge in any cleaning agents."

Finally, clean small areas around the camera lens, attachment ports, or buttons with surface gunk by gently working a dry cotton swab or wooden toothpick around those areas to loosen and remove any buildup.

3. Finish with Disinfecting

You can easily make a cheap and effective cleaning and disinfecting spray for the touchscreens on all your home's electronic devices. As an added cleaning bonus, the distilled water in the recipe keeps mineral deposits off your electronic screens.

ELECTRONICS SCREEN-CLEANING SOLUTION
You'll need:

- A spray bottle
- ½ cup distilled water
- ½ cup isopropyl alcohol
- Microfiber cleaning cloth or other clean lint-free cloth

Pour the distilled water and alcohol into a spray bottle and gently shake to combine. The cleaning solution may be stored in the spray bottle for up to 2 months. Make sure to label and date the spray bottle, so you'll know what's inside and when to use it by.

Spray the cleaning solution lightly onto a clean microfiber cloth and apply it to the screen until it is visibly wet but not dripping. (Never spray cleaners directly on your electronic devices.) Wait 5 minutes for the alcohol to do its disinfecting work, then wipe dry with a clean microfiber cloth. Don't forget to treat the case, too! Allow the phone to air-dry completely—or at least 15 minutes—before replacing the case and powering up.

Remember, to protect your precious touchscreens while getting rid of their collection of germs:

- Don't use an abrasive cloth on electronic screens. Abrasive materials can damage the oleophobic coating; they may also scratch the surface.

- Don't apply pressure when cleaning. The connections between touchscreens and the device's components are ridiculously fragile.

- Apply a screen cleaner to a cloth, not directly on your device. Use the dampened cloth to wipe the screen gently and then use a clean area of the material to buff it dry.

LAPTOPS: NOTEBOOKS LIKE NEW

Laptops are a modern-day godsend. You can use them anywhere. That is also the germy downside to notebooks—they have plenty of opportunities to pick up unsavory characters at every stop: sticky restaurant tables, icky kitchen counters, and unwashed bed linens.

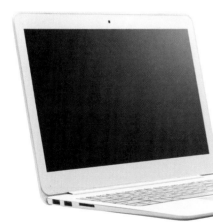

And those questionable surfaces are usually only touching the laptop's outer case. But think about where your hands have been before touching the keyboard!

Ideally, you should clean your laptop weekly to remove bacteria and dust that can cause it to malfunction. Here are the steps to follow.

1. Power Off, Wipe Off

Before cleaning, always turn off the laptop and unplug to ensure it is fully powered off. Electrical currents and liquids don't play well together.

For an exterior cleaning solution, mix a couple drops of liquid dish soap into 2 cups of warm water. Dip a microfiber cloth or other soft lint-free cloth in the soapy mix, then wring until it is just damp, not dripping. With the laptop closed, wipe down the exterior (not the screen yet—that's Step 3) with the cloth. If the case's bottom is grimy, you might need to use a melamine sponge (such as Mr. Clean Magic Eraser) to scour away surface dirt.

Rinse the cloth and wring until just damp, then wipe the laptop case again. Allow to air-dry completely before you turn it on and get back to business.

Avoid getting moisture in any laptop openings. Do not spray liquid directly on your laptop. And don't use aerosol sprays, solvents, abrasives, or cleaners containing hydrogen peroxide that might damage the device's finish.

Stop That Spill

If you spill liquid on your laptop, power down and unplug. Use a dry microfiber cloth to absorb and blot up the moisture. Then turn your keyboard facing down to drain the remaining liquid. Allow your laptop to dry completely before plugging it back in and restarting.

2. Hit the Keyboard

The keyboard is the germiest and dirtiest part of your laptop. Chances are, if you regularly eat over your keyboard, it has picked up some crumbs along the way. Laptop snackers should make cleaning a priority. Skipping cleaning can lead to frequent illnesses from thriving surface bacteria and diminish your laptop's performance.

To tackle keyboard cleaning, dust first by wiping it with a microfiber cloth. Then hold the keyboard upside down over a trash can and gently shake loose any crumbs. Using compressed air, spray the keyboard to remove any leftover crumbs or dust lurking under the keys. Finally, go over the keys with a cotton swab to get inside the crevices and remove any dirt or gunk hiding there.

By the Letter

Laptops enable you to remove an individual keyboard key that may need some extra cleaning. Use a cotton swab and isopropyl alcohol to wipe the entire key and the area beneath it. Allow the key and area to dry for a minute and then replace it.

If your keyboard is particularly dirty, mix a cleaning solution of half isopropyl alcohol and half water. Swab each key using a light circular motion. (Spot test the solution first to ensure the alcohol doesn't remove any of the keyboard letterings.) The alcohol should help cut through the oils left by your fingers while killing any bacteria. Isopropyl alcohol evaporates quickly, so no drying is needed.

3. Clean and Polish the Screen

It's time to give some attention to the screen. Scratches, finger grease, dust, chemicals, and ultraviolet (UV) light can affect your screen's performance and clarity. The surface is coated to make it easier to clean, so you won't need to rub hard to remove fingerprints or oily spots.

To clean LCD screens, use a product tailor-made for the job, sprayed lightly onto a microfiber cloth. For touchscreens, use water or an eyeglass cleaner also applied to a cloth. Wipe the screen with the dampened cloth from top to bottom to remove dust, dirt, and grime.

Important reminders when cleaning any electronic screen:

- Don't use a paper towel to wipe the screen. These and other abrasive materials can cause scratches and leave lint on the screen's surface.

- Never spray anything directly on the screen itself. Liquid drips can get inside the display and cause damage.

- Don't use any type of window cleaner, ammonia, vinegar, or isopropyl alcohol on the screen. It could cause irreversible damage.

4. Check Ports and Vents

Take a look at the ports and cooling vents on the machine to ensure each is free of dust and debris. If not, you can clear them with compressed air. Spray compressed air from an angle so any dust is blown away from an opening, not deeper into it. The fan behind the cooling vents helps keep the laptop from overheating. Spraying an excessive amount of compressed air into the blades can cause them to overspin and damage the fan. Use a light touch here: give the fan a quick blast of air to remove dust and dirt.

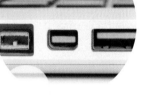

DESKTOP PC: DITCH THE DIRT

One of the best things about a desktop PC is that it doesn't get out much, so it doesn't pick up surface germs on the fly. One of the worst things about a desktop PC is that its sedentary life makes it a natural landing spot for airborne dirt, dust, and germs. Not only is that uninviting to work on, but accumulated dust and dirt can interfere with its performance. Consider giving your computer a quick daily dusting with a microfiber cloth. Once a week, clean the screen and the computer more thoroughly.

Stop! I know what you're thinking. "What's the big deal? Just spray it with a window cleaner, right?" Wrong, computer killer. While it might be the window to your world, your desktop PC is not an actual window, so no Windex. The ammonia in glass cleaners can damage the screens.

It would be best if you didn't spray a cleaner directly on the display or screen at all. Some spray will go through vents and onto the circuit boards. And circuit boards are very finicky about being dropped in on by any liquid, especially strong cleaners. Try this safer method to clean your PC and accessories instead.

1. Power Off, Wipe Off

Don't just power down your computer; turn it off and unplug it to prevent damage or shock. Now that you've taken that safety step, you can move on to cleaning the exterior and tower.

For an exterior cleaning solution, mix 1 part dishwashing liquid to 5 parts lukewarm water. Or mix a solution that's half isopropyl alcohol and half water. Dip a microfiber cloth in your solution of choice and wring well until it is just damp, not dripping. Wipe down the computer's exterior and the tower. A cotton swab dipped in soapy water can be used to clean vents and remove gunk from tight corners.

To remove any remaining soap, wipe with a clean damp cloth. Then dry with a clean cloth.

2. Hit the Keyboard

Ever the efficient one, you double-task a meal and work. The cat hops up for a post–litter box nap. The kids log on, snack in hand, and do their daily homework. No wonder it's covered in germs.

KEYBOARD SPILL SOLUTIONS

Science can't explain it, but all manner of drinks and snacks are attracted to computer keyboards. Here's how to clean up the inevitable mess when it happens:

- Unplug the keyboard.

- If a liquid is spilled, turn the keyboard over and let it drain and dry for at least 24 hours. If the liquid spill was from a sticky drink—a cola or a latte perhaps, pry off the small keycaps with a flathead screwdriver to allow better access to the mess. Take a picture of the keyboard before you remove any keys, to make it easier to put each key back in its rightful home. Don't remove the big keys—the spacebar, the Enter key.

- Clean the keyboard with a slightly damp cotton swab. Gently pry off grimy gunk with a cotton swab dipped in isopropyl alcohol. Allow to dry.

- Rinse the keycaps and allow them to air-dry.

- Replace the keycaps.

- Let everything dry out for at least 24 hours before plugging the keyboard back in and using it.

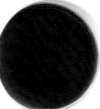

To clean things up, disconnect your keyboard and give it a few good shakes over a trash can to get rid of loose crumbs (and any kitty litter).

Grab a can of compressed air and blow away dust hiding in crevices and between the keys. For dirt or grime on the keys or board frame, wipe with a cloth lightly moistened with a 50-50 solution of isopropyl alcohol and water. Dip a cotton swab in the alcohol solution and clean between each key. (Spot test the solution first to ensure the alcohol doesn't remove any of the keyboard letterings.) Wipe again with a dry cloth.

3. Clean and Polish the Screen
Using a microfiber cloth lightly dampened with distilled water, LCD screen cleaner, or an eyeglass cleaner, gently wipe the screen. If you don't have a microfiber cloth, a coffee filter will work.

4. Decontaminate the Mouse
As you roll a mouse along your desktop, you're also rolling grease, dirt, and gunk into its innards. If not every week, about once a month you need to clean it to keep it rolling along.

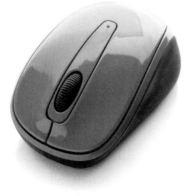

First, power off the mouse, and remove any batteries. If it is wired, unplug it from your computer.

For an optical mouse, gently wipe the lens with a cotton swab dampened with the alcohol solution used earlier. Clean the rubber feet on the bottom to keep your mouse gliding along the same way.

For a mouse with a rolling ball, open the back and remove the ball. Clean the ball with a microfiber cloth dampened in the isopropyl alcohol solution. Gently clean the interior with a cotton swab lightly moistened with the same solution. Allow all the components to air-dry, then reassemble.

5. Check Accessories

Items like a mouse pad or desk blotter can also accumulate dust, grime, and germs. Wipe these surfaces down with a disinfecting wipe. Let dry thoroughly before putting back into place.

REMOTES AND CONTROLLERS: WIN AGAINST GERMS

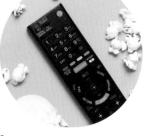

Remote controls and gaming consoles are among the most frequently touched items in our homes. Most TV remotes test positive for the cold virus along with E. coli. That's pretty disgusting when you think about how often we snack in front of the TV while binge-watching our favorite shows.

And, when the remote isn't in your germy hands, it's either on the floor or stuck between the sofa cushions—a cozy dark home that encourages the growth of mold and bacteria. Those remotes and game controllers should be sanitized daily. Here are the steps:

1. Power Down, Dump the Crumbs

Take out the batteries, then replace the cover. Lightly tap the remote, button side down, on a table to dislodge any crumbs from crevices. Use a small brush (a toothbrush works great) to loosen any debris between and around the buttons. Blow off debris carefully with compressed air held at a 75-degree angle; otherwise, you may blow the debris deeper into the keys.

2. Clean the Surface

Go over the surface with a microfiber cloth slightly dampened with a mixture of 1 part water to 1 part isopropyl alcohol. Pay special attention to the buttons and the spaces around them, using a toothpick or your fingernail to remove any stuck-on goo. Game controllers often have built-up dirt and debris in and around the sticks and directional pads.

3. Disinfect and Dry

After cleaning, use a store-bought or DIY disinfectant wipe to clean away germs. Be sure to clean both sides of the remote or game controller thoroughly.

Once the cleaning and disinfecting is complete, allow the device to air-dry completely. Then put the batteries back in, and it's ready to use.

SMART-HOME DEVICES: OFFER YOUR CLEANING HELP

There's no doubt about it: home automation is widespread. Just look at the figures:

- Approximately 9 in 10 U.S. consumers own at least one smart-home device.

- More than 30 percent of those who don't own a connected home device plan on purchasing one in the next year.

- A total of 63 million U.S. homes will likely qualify as "smart" by 2022.

Count me among the smart not-so-few. I'm not so proud of the spaghetti sauce drips on my smart kitchen speaker, however.

Many smart-home devices are "self-learning," meaning that they learn your schedule, behavior, and habits, then adjust themselves accordingly. With my smart speaker in need of a bath, I decided to test that whole "self-learning" thing on my Google Home.

"Hey, Google, clean up your act," I said. "Sorry, I don't understand" came the monotone reply. Not so smart after all, it seems. Sure, it can turn on the lights and play my son's favorite Drake tune on command. But until our smart-home devices get next-generation *really* smart, they are still going to need cleaning help from us if they're to remain presentable in our kitchens and living rooms.

From sticky fingerprints to flying food, these devices can quickly accumulate dirt and grime in high-traffic areas like the kitchen and family room, where they often reside. Whether yours is an Amazon Echo, a Google/Nest device, or some other smart speaker, it could probably use some freshening up. Here's how to bust dust and other gunk lurking on your smart speaker.

Game On!

If your system isn't recognizing a game disc, chances are the surface is soiled. Lightly dampen a clean, lint-free cotton or microfiber cloth. Holding the disc by the rim so that the reflective, non-labeled side is facing up, very gently wipe the surface clean from the center. Wipe lightly again, this time using the cloth's dry area. Place the disc reflective side up on a solid surface to dry for at least 2 minutes before using.

DO

- Unplug your device before performing any cleaning.

- Lightly tap your smart speaker over a trash can to remove surface dust and debris.

- Go over any screen with a screen-cleaning wipe, then tackle the fabric-covered parts with a dry microfiber cloth.

- To clean the mesh fabric, use a lint roller to grab dust and particles sitting on top of the cloth. Run it lightly over the material to avoid pushing dirt and dust deeper into the fabric.

- If there are crumbs or debris stuck in the fabric that the lint roller can't reach, use a vacuum cleaner's attachments to suction out the crud. This should remove nearly all the dust and food stuck in your device.

- If the fabric has a stain, blot the stained area with a slightly damp (not wet) microfiber cloth.

- To clean the plastic parts and touchscreen, and for all-plastic devices like the older-generation Amazon Echos, run a damp microfiber cloth over the surface.

DON'T

- Use isopropyl alcohol, window cleaner, stain removers, or pretty much any liquid that isn't water.

- Use compressed air. (This could damage the drivers.)

- Do not submerge (in a vat of bleach or anything else).

FLAT-SCREEN TVs: CLEAR THE PICTURE

Whether you have a weekly family movie night or just enjoy binge-watching your favorite shows, chances are your television sees a lot of action, so give it its cleaning due. Cleaning your flat-screen TV doesn't require any expensive specialty cleaners. But using the wrong methods or products can void any warranty still in effect. With just a few tools and products, it's a cinch to keep your television screen and its assorted components and accessories clean and dust-free. For clear picture quality and the best performance, television screens should get some attention weekly.

Your first (and last) thought is probably that layer of dust on the screen. When it comes to your entertainment center—whether it's a part of the living room or a whole basement dedicated to TV, gadgets, and gaming—it's essential to go beyond the screen to keep everything clean if you want your expensive equipment to last longer. There are some TV components that, when layered in dust, can affect how well your device works (or doesn't)—like the vents that prevent overheating. Here's how to clean your TV and its essential components safely.

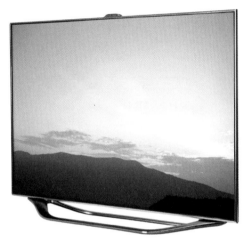

1. Dust the Surface

Before you begin, turn off or unplug your TV. A dark screen makes it easier to spot surface dust.

Use a disposable static-cling duster or microfiber cloth to dust front to back and along the buttons. Don't forget the top, sides, and corners. (Some new televisions come with a cleaning cloth.) If yours is an LCD, make sure you press gently when wiping, as the liquid crystal may get pushed down if you're too vigorous in your cleaning efforts. This can create dark spots. If this should happen, turn it off and on again to fix it.

2. Check the Vents

Make sure the vents are dust-free so that heat can easily escape. On most flat-screen LCD TVs, the vents are at the back. On older TVs, vents may be on the sides and the back. To get the dust out of the vent, put an attachment on your vacuum cleaner and let your vacuum do the work. A duster works for more frequent cleaning, but to ensure you get the dust inside the TV, vacuum at least monthly.

3. Clean the Ports

Ports are where you connect things like HDMI cables, TV-streaming sticks, gaming systems, speakers, and more. If these ports get filled with dust, your TV could have difficulty connecting to external devices. You'll usually find ports on the back, sides, or sometimes beneath or above the TV screen. Instead of reaching for the vacuum here, grab a can of compressed air. When using compressed air, remember not to shake the container and never stick the nozzle inside your TV ports, as the nozzle can damage the sensitive pins in your TV. Hold the nozzle outside the port about an inch away, and spray at an angle so that the air doesn't push dust or debris farther inward.

4. Clear Surface Spots

To remove fingerprints, lightly dampen a clean microfiber cloth with distilled water and gently wipe the grungy surface in circles. Remember to clean the hard-to-reach spots, such as spaces around the TV buttons. For stubborn fingerprints or other resistant grime, lightly spray a microfiber cloth with electronics cleaning spray and wipe clean. Soak up any remaining moisture with a cloth.

5. Let It Dry

Allow all parts of the TV to thoroughly air-dry before switching it back on.

For top TV cleaning results:

- **DO NOT USE AN ABRASIVE CLOTH OR WINDOW CLEANER ON ELECTRONIC SCREENS.** It could damage the oleophobic coating or scratch the surface.

- **USE A LIGHT TOUCH WHEN CLEANING YOUR TELEVISION.** Vigorous scrubbing can cause the screen to crack.

- **APPLY A SCREEN CLEANER TO THE MICROFIBER CLOTH, NOT ON YOUR TELEVISION.** Use the dampened cloth to wipe the screen gently and then use a clean area to buff the surface dry. Never spray any cleaner, including plain water, directly onto any type of flat-screen television. Excessive moisture can permanently damage your screen.

SPEAKERS: SOUND STEPS FOR CLEANING

Speakers tend to sit untouched, not so quietly gathering dirt and grime. If you want your speakers to continue putting out clear-quality sound, make sure to give them some cleaning love the next time you tackle the TV screen and surface.

- Remove the exterior covering (if possible). Check the product manual for guidance if needed.

- To remove dirt on the covering, vacuum using an upholstery brush or other small attachment on a low-suction setting.

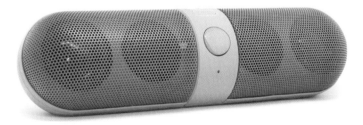

- Use a lint roller to grab and remove any resistant dust.

- Clean any non-fabric areas with a microfiber cloth slightly moistened with water. Clean the entire surface of each speaker thoroughly, refreshing the microfiber cloth as it gets dirty.

- Once cleaning is complete, allow the speakers to air-dry thoroughly, then place the covers back on (if necessary) before using them.

SMARTWATCHES: TIME TO SANITIZE

A smartwatch is a sort of mini computer at your fingertips. It is a fitness tracker and phone and can even replace your bank card for contactless payments. Going to the gym, taking calls, and touching payment terminals can contaminate your wearable. And if you touch your watch without cleaning it, you could be transferring germs to other surfaces—or transferring germs from different surfaces to yourself.

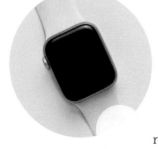

As a result, your smartwatch has the potential to harbor disease-causing microorganisms. Not surprising really, because any item worn close to the skin for long periods is likely to host a variety of skin bacteria. But it does highlight the importance of keeping it—and anything else you regularly wear—as clean as possible.

So, how often should you clean your smartwatch? It's a matter of personal preference. But the longer you wait between cleanings, the more cumbersome the job will likely be. I wipe down the screen daily, wipe down the band once or twice a week, and do a deep clean at least monthly. You don't have to be so finicky. Let's get started!

1. Make a Separation

To clean, first remove the watch band from the main unit to clean it separately. With the band removed, cleaning your smartwatch will be much easier.

2. Clean the Screen

Smartwatch screens require little more than a surface wipe with a dry microfiber cloth. If you don't have a microfiber cloth or a lot of dirt and grime isn't coming off, you can use a new coffee filter lightly dampened with water. Don't use a paper towel; these can leave lint on the screen. Gently wipe the screen with the filter, and

Go Straight to the Source

To keep your personal electronics adequately cleaned and disinfected, it's essential to follow manufacturer guidelines. If unavailable, follow the steps outlined on these pages to clean and disinfect the devices.

fingerprints or grime should come right off. Pay close attention to where the heart-rate sensor touches your skin; dirt and oils can build up here relatively easily and quickly. To remove the gunk, use a wooden toothpick or a toothbrush to nudge it out.

If all else fails, add 1 teaspoon of rubbing alcohol to ½ cup of water; dip a microfiber cloth, coffee filter, or soft-bristled toothbrush in it; and gently wipe the screen again. Make sure to rinse the seating area where the watch band normally sits.

Avoid any holes or openings on your watch; liquid that gets inside could harm the device. And never use chemical solvents on your electronic screens. No Windex. No 409 spray. If your watch is water-resistant, you can get it wet to clean it, even dunk it in a very diluted bath of water and liquid soap (about one drop

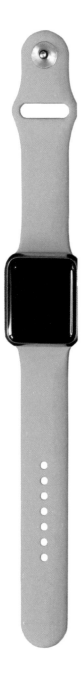

of soap per cup of water). Blot-rinse with water and a clean cloth or rag to remove any soapy residue. Then dry with a fresh cloth or rag.

3. Clean the Band

How you clean your band depends entirely on the material of which it is made. But for all band types, start your cleaning routine by wiping the band lint-free with a lightly dampened cloth.

SILICONE, NYLON, AND METAL WATCH BANDS can be submerged in water for cleaning. Put a small amount of soap (dishwashing or handwashing) into a bowl or stopped-up sink of water. Use your fingers to work out any dirt or lint. Metal watch bands can be harder to clean because they have many chain links and other crevices where grime can hide. However, you have options. For stubborn grime or dried-on dirt, a quick pass with a soft-bristled toothbrush or wooden toothpick will help to loosen and remove the gunk. Rinse the band in water and let it air-dry thoroughly.

To sanitize these types of watch bands, dampen a microfiber cloth (or use an alcohol-based disinfectant wipe) with an electronics screen cleaner (see page 93) and thoroughly wipe down both sides of the watch band. Isopropyl alcohol evaporates quickly, so there's no need to rinse the band when you're done. The alcohol kills the bacteria that can cause your watch band to smell and any other microbes that could make you sick.

LEATHER BANDS are far more finicky and shouldn't be submerged in water. Apple recommends spot cleaning leather with a soft damp cloth and then letting it dry completely. Of course, water won't disinfect a leather watch band (or anything else).

While you can't disinfect it, you can clean it with a leather cleaner and conditioner. Conditioning does double duty—it both cleans and protects it. I use a brand called KIWI Outdoor Saddle Soap. It's ideal for removing dirt and grime on all leather types. Always test a small part of the leather first with the conditioner to make sure it doesn't cause any color changes.

Remove surface dirt with a brush or cloth. Then apply a small dab of leather conditioner to a cloth or sponge. Rub it on the surface, wait a few minutes for it to dry, then buff the same spot with a clean cloth or sponge. If you don't see any color or texture changes, clean the rest of the band the same way.

When your smartwatch is clean and dry, wash your hands up to the wrist, just above where the watch rests, and dry them. Now you're ready to reassemble your wearable tech and put it back on.

FITNESS TRACKERS: FAST TRACK TO CLEAN

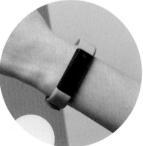

Like smartwatches, fitness trackers are designed to be worn for more extended periods and for exercising. So, no surprise here, they get sweaty. A quick rinse in the shower is a good start, but that won't kill germs or remove more stubborn dirt and stuck-on grime where disease-causing microorganisms love to take up residence.

That's why you should clean your fitness tracker regularly, especially after a workout. Fitbit offers specific recommendations for cleaning its fitness trackers, and like Apple's, these recommendations include using isopropyl alcohol to disinfect the devices. Fitbit also recommends avoiding soap-based cleansers that can get trapped in the band and cause skin irritation. Instead, the company recommends soap-free cleaners and thoroughly rinsing the devices to wash away surface dirt.

HEADPHONES AND EARBUDS: PROTECT YOUR EARS

Smartwatches and fitness trackers aren't the only wearables that need cleaning regularly. Earbuds and headphones need some cleaning TLC, too. Whether yours are over-ear or in-ear headphones, cleaning off lingering earwax and surface disinfecting aren't only good practices for hygienic reasons. They may even improve the sound quality.

If you use your headphones while working out, sweat can build up in the ear cups and cause them to start smelling bad. In addition, a buildup of earwax can clog the drivers and reduce not only the volume but also the clarity of the sound.

Listen Up

While clean earbuds will protect your ears against infection, these tips will help prevent hearing damage:

- Jam your workout, watch a movie, or play video games at no louder than 60 percent of the max volume.

- Try to limit your daily time with earbuds inserted to 60 minutes. If you need to go longer for work or school purposes, take frequent breaks.

A study by SeniorLiving.org found that aside from being coated in sweat and wax (gross but true), the average pair of personal in-ear headphones is home to 119,186 CFU, or colony-forming units—more than 2,700 times the bacteria on an average cutting board and 330 times more bacteria than on a kitchen countertop. Not all headphones in the study were crawling with germs, however. One pair had a CFU count of 20; another tipped the scales at 830,000 CFU. Even with such a wide range and the possibility of your headphones falling toward the lower end, researchers concluded that it can't hurt to disinfect them every so often.

Common bacteria that can live on your earbuds include *Staphylococcus* that can cause a painful ear infection. Then there's all the dirt, bacteria, and other microbes you can't see that might make you sick. Studies have shown that headphone use increases bacterial growth inside the ear. Clean headphones are just more sanitary.

Cleaning Over-Ear Headphones

How you clean your over-ear headphones will vary. Many brands are designed for easy cleaning, with removable ear cups and cables that unplug at both ends. If yours are not so cleaning-friendly, you'll need to be careful not to damage them. Consult the manufacturer's cleaning instructions, if available.

To clean and sanitize over-ear headphones, you'll need:
- Electronics cleaning solution (page 93)
- Disposable (or regular) microfiber cloth
- Cotton swabs

If you have concerns about damaging any fabric on your headphones, test any cleaning solution on an inconspicuous area first.

- Start by removing the ear cups from the headphones (if possible) to more easily access the mesh below.

- To de-germify, grab the electronics cleaning solution you made for your phone (page 93), spray it lightly on a disposable (or regular) microfiber cloth, and wipe away stuck-on grime, bacteria, and other nasties from both ear cups and the rest of the headphones.

- Lightly spray a cotton swab with cleaning solution and work it into any nooks and crannies (i.e., areas like fabric folds) on both ear cups.

- Extend the headphones as far as possible and wipe the exterior and any buttons, volume dials, or remotes you use with a microfiber cloth dampened with cleaning spray. Spend some extra cleaning time on the area where you grip the headphones while putting them on and taking them off.

- To clean the mesh on the main speakers, dab a cloth or cotton swab with cleaning solution and wipe. If your headphones have a microphone (like a gaming headset, for example), clean the mesh and adjustable arm with the cleaning solution, too.

- Wipe down any cables, including the rubber grip near the jack, with a microfiber cloth dampened with cleaning solution.

- Allow the headphone components to air-dry completely before you reassemble and use your headphones.

Cleaning In-Ear Headphones

In-ear headphones are generally less hygienic because you actually put them inside your ear. Some sit quite deep in your ear canal to form a seal, thanks to their silicone tips. While the sound is superior, the risk of getting an ear infection is greater with these devices.

To clean and sanitize in-ear headphones, you'll need:
- Individual isopropyl alcohol wipes
- Wooden toothpicks
- Blu-Tack (or similar adhesive putty)
- Cotton swabs
- Isopropyl alcohol
- Paper towels or microfiber cloths
- Electronics cleaning solution (page 93)

If your in-ear headphones have removable silicone ear tips, remove and clean them separately after each use, being careful not to tear the silicone.

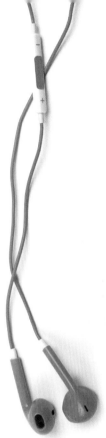

- Clean the surface and the interior holes of each ear tip with an isopropyl alcohol wipe.

- To remove earwax in the holes, work it free with a toothpick. To disinfect, wrap a toothpick in an alcohol wipe, and carefully work it around each hole. Afterward, set them somewhere safe to air-dry.

- To clean the grille parts, gently press some Blu-Tack (or similar adhesive putty) along the speaker mesh. Pull quickly to remove any dirt or wax, then repeat until the speaker mesh is clean. To disinfect the speaker mesh, dip a cotton swab in rubbing alcohol and use it to wipe down the surface thoroughly. This should also help loosen any remaining grime for easy removal. Clean speaker mesh is not only more sanitary; it may improve the sound quality, too.

- To clean the drivers entirely, dampen a paper towel or clean microfiber cloth with the electronics cleaning solution (page 93) and clean around any sensors (like the ear-detection sensors on Apple AirPods).

- Wipe down cables, remotes, or the rubber grip near the jack with a clean cloth lightly damped with cleaning spray. Allow the alcohol solution to evaporate before you store or wear your in-ear headphones. Alcohol dries quickly, so you shouldn't have to wait more than 60 seconds.

Cleaning Headphone Cases

When cleaning your headphone case, remember to remove surface dirt and grime before you disinfect it. Bacteria and other pathogens can cling to grime, even after you clean the case.

For over-ear headphone cases, spot clean with soap and water, but take care not to saturate the surface. Isopropyl alcohol can disinfect the fabric, but spot test first to make sure the alcohol won't discolor it.

Some wireless in-ear headphones come with a charging case. It's essential to clean these, too. Otherwise, your now germ-free headphones will just get germy again the next time you tuck them away. For AirPods or similar headphones, use a soft-bristled toothbrush to dislodge built-up grime around the lid hinge. To disinfect inside the case, use a cotton swab dipped in isopropyl alcohol to clean any hard-to-reach charging bays.

Keeping your electronics gadgets clean and sanitized isn't that difficult, after all! It just requires knowing the safest sanitizing solution for each tech type. And, by regularly sanitizing your tech toys, you're not only helping to keep yourself healthy, but you're also helping to protect the health of those you encounter daily.

IF YOU'RE A FAN OF FANS

Window fans, ceiling fans, and those on stands have the tendency to collect airborne dust and grease over time and with frequent use. Fans may also spread airborne human pathogens. To be on the safe side—and because dust- and grime-free fan blades don't move the air around as efficiently—it makes sense to give your fans some cleaning attention. Grab a pillowcase for a super-helpful tool to capture and hold dust and grime.

- Start by turning the fan off and unplugging as needed. For fans other than ceiling fans, remove grilles to access the blades.

- Use a pillowcase to wipe down and clean the downrod, motor housing, and canopy of ceiling fans. Clean grilles of other types of fans with soap and water in the sink, then allow the parts to dry.

- Next, move to the fan's blades. Gently slide the pillowcase over the top of each blade. Press gently to remove dirt and grime, then remove the pillowcase. Continue until all are free of dust and grime.

- Reassemble any dry parts as needed.

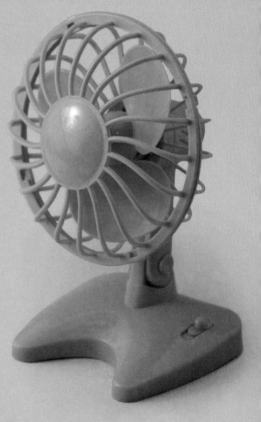

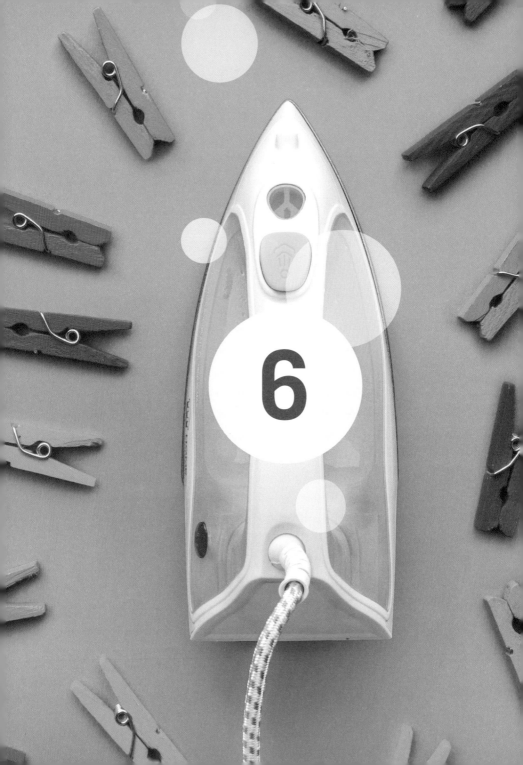

A CLEAN LAUNDRY ROOM

Steps to Safe Handling & Disinfection

DURING COLD AND FLU SEASON, or when someone in your home is ill, disinfecting laundry and handling it safely without spreading illness is super important but can feel challenging. You know how (mostly) to get rid of the usual suspects—the ground-in grunge and grime. But how do you disinfect clothes, and avoid spreading germs all over the house and not get sick in the process?

Honestly, with all we know about germs these days, it's smart to take handling of worn clothing seriously with laundry precautions every day—not just when a virus hits your household. It's not a bad idea to ditch your clothing and anything that may have hitched to it after any time you expose yourself to the wide world of germs out there. Treat yourself to fresh duds before you settle in on the sofa. But resist the urge to toss the day's dirty duds on the bedroom chair or the bed. To corral germs, give worn clothes their own bin or hamper to rest in until wash day rolls around.

When it's time to hit the laundry room, there's no need for the wash day blues. You can get the wash done and keep you and your home safe in the process. The best approach combines safe laundry handling and easy-to-use laundry additives and other methods of disinfecting laundry to avoid the spread of illness.

DISINFECTING YOUR WASHER AND DRYER

Before you gather up those dirty duds and head to the laundry room, take a moment to sanitize the space, particularly the washer and dryer. The condition of your washer and dryer plays a significant role in the cleanliness of your clothing.

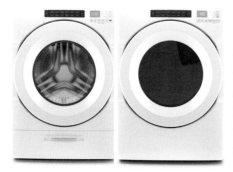

Clean your washer weekly with an easy vinegar treatment. Then call out the heavier arsenal to disinfect your washing machine monthly—or at least semi-annually—to kill germs that may have taken up residence there. If a virus cycles through your home, jump in with some ASAP disinfection.

Washer Cleaning Routine

To control germs in your washer, run a full cycle using hot water at the maximum fill setting once a week. Add 2 cups of distilled white vinegar after the machine fills. Do not launder any clothing or add detergent during this cycle. Its purpose is to dissolve residue and kill germs in the machine and drain.

Washer Disinfecting Steps

Disinfect the washing machine monthly or immediately after washing the clothes of someone who is sick. A surprising number of hardy germs can survive a warm-water swim. You should also disinfect it after running a load of clothes contaminated with poison oak or poison ivy, pesticides, or petroleum chemicals.

Disinfecting is especially important if you regularly wash in cold water. Washing machines collect dirt, grime, and bacteria from your clothes, towels, and bedding. If you only use cold water, residual buildup of laundry detergent and fabric softener can trap and hold germs and bacteria in a washing machine. These buggers can transfer back to your clothes, causing odor and potentially spreading disease. Here's how to sanitize your washing machine using chlorine bleach.

CLEAN CHOICES
Options Beyond Bleach

If you don't like to use bleach, disinfectant alternatives include pine oil, phenolic disinfectants, or quaternary (quats) disinfectants to clean your washer. Do not use oxygen or "color-safe" bleach; it is not a certified disinfectant. Read and follow the usage directions on product labels and follow the same steps as for cleaning with chlorine bleach. Choose one cleaner only; never mix cleaning chemicals.

1. Set the washer's water temperature to hot. If your washing machine has a sanitizing cycle, use it. Otherwise, choose a heavy-duty or cotton setting.

2. Add 1 cup of bleach to the washer drum (both front-load and top-load models). Do not add any clothes.

3. Run a full cycle.

4. When the cycle is complete, check inside the washer and especially under the lid and near any rubber seals for signs of mold or residual detergent. If you find any grime, scrub the area with a soft-bristled brush and a diluted bleach solution (i.e., 4 teaspoons of bleach added to 1 quart of water).

5. Remove all dispensers (detergent, bleach, and fabric softener) and filters, and wash them in the sink in warm soapy water. Rinse, dry completely, and replace.

6. Run another rinse cycle to ensure that all bleach is removed before doing a load of laundry.

7. Clean the exterior. Wipe the top, front, and sides clean with a solution of chlorine bleach and hot water. Don't forget any knobs. Rinse and dry with a soft cloth. Use an electronics disinfecting wipe on any control panels.

Dryer Duty

To control germs in your dryer, clean the inside of the drum and the door with a disinfecting wipe or bleach solution once a week. You should also disinfect it after running a load of clothes contaminated with poison oak or poison ivy, pesticides, or petroleum chemicals.

Routine maintenance should include emptying the lint screen after each load. But even if you consistently clear the lint screen, particles can accumulate at other places along the exhaust system—as fine as your lint screen is, some lint particles will still be finer. One early tip-off to a clogged vent: your clothes don't seem to dry in one cycle. Rather than risk a fire, plan to check the venting system every six months.

Be sure to wait until the dryer is completely cool to follow these disinfecting steps.

Be a Natural Softy

You can have soft, fluffy clothes and thirsty towels without having to endure the waxy after-effects of chemical fabric softeners. Instead, add 1 cup of white vinegar (a bit more for large loads) to the fabric softener dispenser, so it's added to the final rinse water. The acidity will dissolve detergent residue that can make clothes and towels feel rough.

1. Remove the lint screen. Clear it of any lint buildup, then soak the filter in the sink in warm soapy water.

2. Ready a cleaning solution. Add 4 teaspoons of chlorine bleach to 1 quart of water. Or use pine oil, phenolic disinfectant, or quaternary disinfectant, following label instructions.

3. Wipe the dryer drum. Dip a soft cloth into the cleaning solution. Wipe the surface of the dryer drum, the rubber seals and gaskets, and the interior of the dryer door, using enough solution to make surfaces visibly wet. Let sit for at least 10 minutes.

4. Return to the lint screen. While your disinfectant solution is doing its work on the dryer drum, go back to your soaking lint screen. Rinse it, shake off excess moisture, then allow it to air-dry.

5. Rinse the drum well with a cloth dipped in water. Then wipe the drum dry with a clean cloth or allow it to air-dry.

6. Clean the exterior. Wipe down the outside of the dryer, including any knobs, handles, and the door, with the cleaning solution. Use an electronics disinfecting wipe on any control panels. Let sit for at least 10 minutes. Rinse well with a cloth dipped in water. Allow it to air-dry or buff dry.

7. Replace the lint screen once thoroughly dry.

No More Icky Iron

Although it doesn't need the regular attention your washer and dryer do, your iron benefits from a little TLC at least a few times a year. You can use a commerical cleaner, following label directions. But the cleaners you already have at home can tackle the job just as well in most cases.

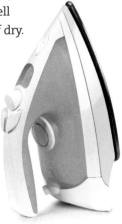

CHECKLISTS FOR A CLEAN LAUNDRY ROOM

The laundry room is the house's workhorse. It's a fundamental part of housekeeping, and an area that needs to remain clean and organized to function properly. If you're not giving your laundry room the attention it needs to stay in tip-top working order, use this list to set up a cleaning weekly, monthly, and seasonal schedule.

WEEKLY

- Dust ceilings and walls.
- Dust windows, doors, and baseboards.
- Disinfect switch plates and doorknobs.
- Wipe clean washer and dryer.
- Sweep or vacuum floors.

MONTHLY

- Disinfect the washing machine.
- Disinfect the dryer.
- Sanitize the trash can.
- Clean the utility sink.
- Sweep and mop behind the washer and dryer.

SEASONALLY (SPRING AND FALL)

- Wash the windows.
- Deep clean the window treatments.
- Clean the iron.
- Clean the dryer vent.

Grab the dish detergent. One of the best ways to clean an iron just might be the simplest. Add a few drops of liquid dish detergent to a bowl or bucket of water. Dip a clean cloth in the solution and wipe your iron's cool soleplate (i.e., iron's undersurface).

Freshen with vinegar. Making sure to use the distilled white variety, dampen a clean cloth and wipe the (cool) iron's soleplate to remove any gunk. If residue remains, soak a clean towel in the vinegar, then lay the iron's soleplate on the towel for 15 to 30 minutes. Wipe clean and rub dry.

To clean out the iron's steam vents, dip a cotton swab in your soap solution or the distilled vinegar. Then use the damp cotton swab to scrub those holes.

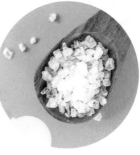

Battle stains with salt. Nasty stains that won't disappear? Place parchment paper on your ironing board, then spread salt across the paper. With the iron on a low-heat setting, move the soleplate across the salted paper using a firm motion. Let the iron cool, then wipe clean.

To prevent buildup and odor, remember to empty the water reservoir after every use.

HOW TO HANDLE LAUNDRY SAFELY

Whether you're going about your weekly wash routine or safeguarding your household with extra sanitizing during a virus outbreak, some simple steps can help you avoid germ transfer as you tackle handling all those loads of laundry.

- Wear gloves when handling dirty laundry. Disposable gloves are best for this task. If you prefer reusable gloves, don't wear them while cleaning the rest of the house. When the laundry is all set and in process, launder the gloves to disinfect them as well.

- Wash your hands after handling laundry. It's a simple step that we often forget. Even if you've been wearing gloves, it's still necessary.

- Avoid shaking dirty laundry—it will send any germs spiraling into the air. And don't "hug" laundry close to your body. Do whatever you can to reduce contact with possibly contaminated items.

- Disinfect laundry baskets and hampers regularly. Use separate containers for clean and dirty laundry. It can help to place washable or disposable liners in laundry baskets and hampers. Plan to clean the insides with a disinfecting wipe or spray or a bleach solution (make sure to rinse!) after use.

- Don't forget to wipe down any surfaces you used to sort—like the top of the washer and dryer or nearby counters. Zap them with those disinfecting wipes.

SANITIZING SURPRISE
Good News for Procrastinators

If you can't get to that dirty laundry right away, it's okay—as long it's safely contained and untouched in a hamper. In fact, just a couple of days can give time for any pathogens to die off the surface.

HOT, WARM, OR COLD?

When it's time to select a laundry-wash setting and temperature, let your fabrics determine the cycle: jeans and heavy items get the normal or regular cycle; sheer and delicate fabrics do best in a gentle cycle; and so on, according to the label.

How important is the right wash water temperature? It directly affects how well your laundry detergent (and any disinfecting or sanitizing additives) clean, and it also affects the life span of your clothes. So, here again, it's important to follow the care labels. If a label is not legible, remember that hot water works well on ground-in and hard-to-remove dirt on sturdy fabrics. Still, few labels recommend regular hot-water washing.

Hot Water

Use hot water to sanitize seriously soiled clothes (gardening or children's clothing) and to regularly disinfect clothes, dish towels, washcloths, bath towels, bedding, and pillowcases. Generally speaking, whites, very dirty or greasy clothes, and sturdy colorfast fabrics that retain their dye can be washed in hot water. (Whites warrant the solo treatment, no matter what the temperature.)

Fast Colorfastness Test

How can you tell if an item is "colorfast"? Do the cotton swab test. Place the inner seam of a shirt or sweater on a paper towel, then soak a cotton swab with cool water and press down firmly on the seam. If no color appears on the swab, it's colorfast and safe to wash.

Warm Water

Warm temperature minimizes color fading and wrinkling. Choose it to wash regular and sturdy fabrics, towels, jeans, cottons, sheets, sturdy playwear, school uniforms, 100 percent manmade fibers, and moderately soiled stuff.

Cold Water

Use cold water for dark or bright colors that may run or fade; delicate fabrics, including washable silk, swimsuits, and active wear; and delicate lingerie. Cold water will minimize the shrinking of washable woolens. It's also okay for lightly soiled clothes.

Always use cold water for clothes stained with blood, wine, or coffee. Warm water could set these stains. A cold-water rinse saves the energy used per load by up to one-third and minimizes wrinkling in synthetic or permanent-press fabrics.

CLOTHES CAPTIONING: LAUNDRY LABELS

The Federal Trade Commission (FTC) requires manufacturers and importers to attach a label with proper care instructions to garments. They will be either solely symbols, or symbols and words. Clothing care labels tell you all you need to know about how to wash, dry, and iron your favorite dress or work uniform. Read your clothing care label: it's the secret to successful laundry. After all, we've all heard those stories of ruined silk thought to be washable or that wool sweater that came out of the dryer three sizes too small. Here's how to decipher what you see, along with a shortcut chart at right.

Washing Method

A clean tub-like icon means safe to machine wash. Hands in the tub? Hand-wash is recommended. If the tub is crossed out, the item can't be washed. Circle? Dry-clean. If the circle is crossed out, dry-cleaning is not an option.

Washing Temperature

A tub-like icon with dots tells you the recommended wash temperature. Translate as one dot for cool/cold, two for warm, three for hot.

Washing Cycle

Any lines indicated under that tub guide you to the appropriate wash cycle. No lines? That's normal cycle. One line is a recommendation for permanent press, and two lines means delicate/gentle.

LAUNDRY AT A GLANCE

WASHING SYMBOLS

Machine wash	Machine wash, permanent press	Machine wash, delicate	Hand wash	Do not wash	Do not wring
Water temperature 30°C	Water temperature 40°C	Water temperature 50°C	Water temperature 60°C	Water temperature 70°C	Water temperature 95°C

DRYING SYMBOLS

Tumble dry	Low heat	Medium heat	High heat	Dry flat	Dry in the shade
No heat	Permanent press	Delicate	Hang to dry	Drip dry	Do not tumble dry
Short cycle	Reduced moisture	Low heat	No steam finishing	Do not dry-clean	Do not wet clean

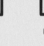

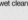

IRONING SYMBOLS

Low temperature	Medium temperature	High temperature	Iron	Do not iron	No steam

BLEACHING SYMBOLS

Any solvent	Any solvent except tetrachlorethylene	Petroleum solvent only	Wet cleaning	Nonchlorine bleach	Do not bleach

Drying Method

Dryer symbols, often shown as a square with a circle in the middle, indicate that tumble dry is allowed. But watch for warnings that drying is not recommended—that dryer icon crossed out. Seeing other symbols? A square that resembles an envelope indicates line dry. A square with a bisecting horizontal line means dry the item flat. A crossed-out twisted symbol (looking almost like an old-fashioned wrapped candy) lets you know you shouldn't wring out this piece of clothing or damage may occur.

Drying Temperature

If machine drying is an option, the circle inside the dryer square will guide you to a temperature setting. Empty circle? Any choice of heat is fine—you're home-free. Three dots inside the dryer circle recommend high heat; two dots is a vote for medium heat; one dot is a warning to stick with low heat. Filled-in circle? Skip any type of heat in favor of air-drying.

Bleaching Instructions

A triangle is the bleach symbol. A triangle intact lets you know that bleaching is allowed. If it's crossed out, put the bleach away. A triangle with stripes communicates you can use nonchlorine bleach only.

Ironing Guidance

Check for the iron symbol. If it's completely crossed out, ironing could damage this particular piece. Lower extending lines crossed out? That's just a caution to avoid steam. If you've got a go to iron, the dots on the iron indicate the recommended temperature: one dot for low heat, two for medium, and three for high.

THE DIRT ON DETERGENTS

Your everyday laundry detergent should be a tough all-fabric cleaner that works as well on grungy gardening duds as it does on collared polo shirts.

How much detergent should you use? Reading product labels is a good starting point. The best amount depends on the hardness of your water (i.e., the harder the water, the more detergent needed), how dirty the clothing is (i.e., more soil requires more detergent), and the wash water temperature (i.e., cooler water requires more detergent). Your machine style (i.e., front- versus top-loader) also affects your detergent needs—make sure you know your manufacturer's recommendation.

Detergent works by loosening soil in fabrics. The removed dirt is then held in the wash water until drained. If you notice greasy-looking stains and gunk building up on the outer tub of the washer, you might be using too little detergent. These soils can then wash off and redeposit on other loads. When you notice the ick, clean the machine and adjust your detergent amount for future loads.

Ready, Set, Wash

- Check clothing labels for care recommendations.

- Separate whites from colors to keep dyes from bleeding onto lighter-colored fabrics.

- Separate heavily soiled items from lightly soiled clothes, so you can wash very dirty items on their own.

- Use the recommended detergent amount (per the label), but adjust if soil, water, or machine conditions are not average.

SANITIZING YOUR LAUNDRY

Simply putting your household's clothing in the washing machine with laundry detergent may leave it looking cleaner and brighter, but it isn't going to get rid of those germs. You might think that all that agitating would kill viruses, bacteria, and fungi, but it just isn't enough. You have to disinfect laundry to truly sanitize it.

Getting Started

The only real wild card in the laundry sanitizing process is which disinfectant to use. But the start and finish steps are essentially the same:

- **ALWAYS CHOOSE THE WARMEST WATER TEMPERATURE SAFE FOR THE FABRIC.** That's the official CDC recommendation. Heat helps to disinfect, especially in combination with household disinfectants, such as bleach.

- **CONSIDER USING A LAUNDRY DETERGENT THAT CONTAINS BLEACH,** as appropriate. Read the product label description and guidelines to avoid ruining your favorite T-shirt or pair of jeans. Another option is soaking clothes in a solution containing quaternary ammonium before washing to boost the disinfecting power on wash day. We'll dive more into disinfectant choices in the next section.

- **MAKE SURE LAUNDRY DRIES THOROUGHLY.** If your fabric can handle high heat, that's great. If not, dry it on the highest appropriate setting. Or consider letting it air-dry in sunlight. But whatever you do, avoid putting away (or wearing) moist clothing, as it becomes a breeding ground for germs.

> **SANITIZING SURPRISE**
> **Laundry**
> **Social Distancing**
>
> Don't overload your washer. If clothes are packed too tightly, they won't circulate freely in the wash water and won't get completely clean—or sanitized.

Laundry Disinfectant Choices

No matter what sanitizer you choose, follow the product's directions to the letter and use only the recommended amount of disinfectant. Here is some information that can help you decide what may be right for the range of clothing in your household's closets and drawers.

CHLORINE BLEACH is the ultimate multitasker that you probably already have in your household's cleaning supply. It keeps clothes white longer and cleans and protects surfaces. Disinfecting bleach kills 99.9 percent of germs and kills norovirus, flu virus, E. coli, Salmonella, and more. Flexible to be used in any temperature water, chlorine bleach is an effective disinfectant for white clothes and some colored garments.

- Top-loaders: Before adding clothes, pour ½ cup of bleach into the machine along with your usual laundry detergent. Wait for the water to fill before adding your clothes.

- Front-loaders: Simply place in the machine's bleach dispenser.

PHENOLIC DISINFECTANTS, such as Lysol Laundry Sanitizer, are fairly odorless laundry sanitizers that contain no bleach and kill 99 percent of bacteria like Staphylococcus aureus and Klebsiella pneumoniae. They are gentle on fabrics, can be used on whites and colors, and work even in cold water.

- Top-loaders: Add 2 capfuls to the fabric softener dispenser at the start of the laundry cycle or during the rinse. If your machine doesn't have a fabric softener dispenser, add directly to the drum of the machine during the rinse cycle.

- Front-loaders: Add 2 capfuls to the fabric softener compartment at the start of the laundry cycle.

PINE OIL DISINFECTANTS, such as Pine-Sol and Lestoil, can disinfect whites as well as colored fabrics that chlorine bleach would damage. Disinfectants must contain at least 80 percent pine oil to destroy germs. Pine oil is toxic to cats, however, so do not use it if you have feline family members.

- Top-loaders: Add 1 cup to the machine while the water is filling the washer, then add clothes. Run a second rinse cycle to remove any lingering scent.

- Front-loaders: Add to the machine's fabric softener dispenser. Run a second rinse cycle to remove any lingering scent.

QUATERNARY DISINFECTANTS, such as GermBloc, are effective in warm and cold water. Add during the rinse cycle because prolonged exposure can damage some fabrics. Quats can be tougher than other laundry sanitizers to find at the store.

- Top-loaders: Add per label directions during the rinse cycle.

- Front-loaders: Fill the fabric softener dispenser per label directions.

VINEGAR. Distilled white vinegar has some disinfecting properties that can be combined with heat drying for additional disinfection. Do not substitute apple cider vinegar or white vinegar, which may stain clothing.

- Top-loaders: Add 2 cups during the rinse cycle. The vinegar smell will dissipate during the cycle.

- Front-loaders: Fill the fabric softener dispenser with ¾ cup of distilled white vinegar.

POWER FROM YOUR DRYER OR STEAMER

Okay, let's assume you're having a really bad day. You didn't feel up to stopping for a quick bleach run on the way home, but you have some dirty laundry that really needs attention.

If you don't have a laundry sanitizing product handy, wash your clothes as usual, then pop everything in the dryer for at least 45 minutes. Ample heat through the dry cycle can fight a meaningful attack against nasty germs.

But being the savvy launderer you are, you take a peek at your new shirt's label and—oh no! Seems that blouse can't go in the regular wash and dry. Now what? No problem, you've got this! When clothes can't handle machine drying, or you need to disinfect a garment in a pinch, your steamer can help. Steam on its own is an effective sanitizer for clothes and other linens. Don't have a dedicated steamer? Use your iron for the same thing. Just spritz the garment with water, then set your iron to the cotton or linen setting. Clean clothing crisis averted!

WASH DAY PRIORITIES CHECKLIST

- Wash sheets weekly in warm or hot water to keep linens fresh.

- Wash bath towels and bath mats weekly. Damp towels are bacterial breeding grounds and, truth be told, plenty of people still aren't washing their hands correctly.

- Change dish towels daily; wash weekly.

- Replace bathroom hand towels daily and any time they feel damp; wash weekly.

Now that your regular household laundry pile is under control and your laundry space is sanitized, it's to time to learn how to ramp up all your clean freak efforts when someone in the household is sick.

STAYING SAFE AT THE LAUNDROMAT

If you use a pay-as-you-go washer and dryer, you may not want to spend additional money or time running an empty disinfecting load. But that doesn't mean you need to expose your laundry to the risk of a carryover infection. These seven steps can help keep you and your laundry safe.

1. Before using a machine, wipe the buttons, knobs, handles, and door with a disinfecting wipe.

2. Avoid using shared laundry carts.

3. If you can get away with using just a single machine, wash your towels for the first load, using the hottest and longest machine cycle. Add bleach or another laundry disinfectant. Use this machine for the rest of your laundry if possible.

4. If using several machines, add a disinfecting laundry product to each load.

5. Before using a dryer, wipe the interior with a disinfecting wipe until it is visibly wet. Allow the disinfectant to dry for about 5 minutes before use. Use this dryer for the remainder of your laundry if possible.

6. Wash your hands after you've finished doing laundry.

7. Once home, disinfect the interior and exterior of your laundry hamper or basket with a disinfecting spray or wipe.

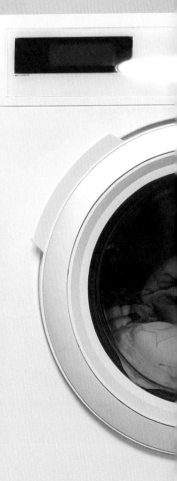

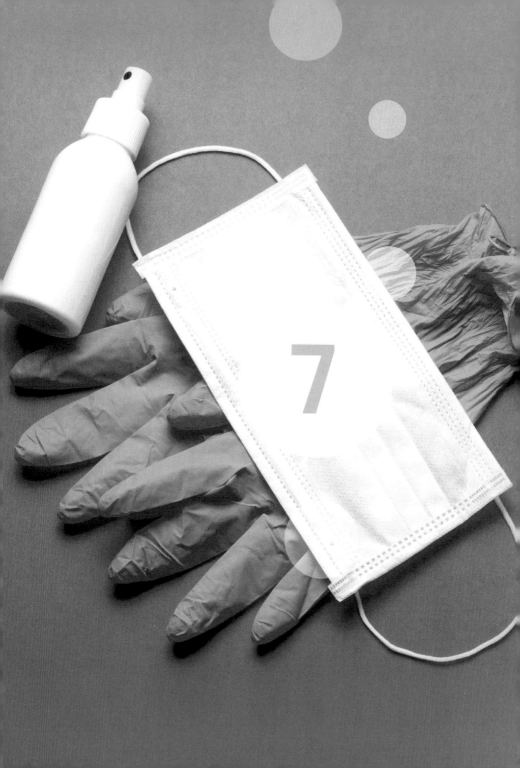

WHEN SOMEONE IS SICK

How to Take Care & Keep Everyone Safe

WHEN SOMEONE IN YOUR HOME IS SICK, you can expect many facets of your daily routine to undergo some changes, including how you clean your house. How often you disinfect surfaces, launder pillowcases, and even where you eat dinner could be factors that determine whether others in the household stay healthy or you take to a sickbed yourself.

No matter how much you love someone, chances are, you don't want to share their flu or cold virus or any other infectious diseases, for that matter. Living with and caring for a sick child or partner means knowing how not to get sick yourself.

It's all about risk mitigation. You can't eliminate the risk entirely, but you can minimize it. When you do that, you're stacking the odds in your favor—of not getting sick, that is. When anyone in your home is exhibiting the telltale signs of a cold, flu, or any type of contagious illness, priority number one is to prevent the disease from spreading to others in the home.

Without timely action on your part, if left unchecked, viral transmission can ricochet through your home at breakneck speed. One recent study found that family members of people who had the flu and eventually got sick began showing symptoms within a mere 2.9 days of the first household diagnosis.

Beyond washing your hands frequently and correctly, daily surface cleaning and disinfecting is your best defense. Flu viruses live on hard surfaces for up to 24 hours. Norovirus is frequently blamed for stomach bugs and can linger on surfaces for days or weeks. Other viruses can live on hard surfaces for up to two weeks. Knowing how to destroy these hardy germs can keep sickness from spreading in your home. So, it's time to learn how to take care of yourself and keep everyone safe while getting your loved one healthy.

DESIGNATE RECOVERY SPACE

They're probably not going to like it, but this first step is one of the most important: create sick rooms. To limit exposure to others residing in the household, designate "sick rooms"—a bedroom and bathroom just for the ill person's use. Then make sure everyone else uses others. Encourage your sick family member to stay separated from other household members as much as possible.

Flu and other viruses spread when the sick person coughs, sneezes, or even talks, affecting people as far away as six feet. Germs also spread when you touch a surface that has viruses on it. You'll want to nip this one in the bud by changing up your daily routine so that it includes enough time for you to spend on disinfecting surface patrol.

Yes, I know it's hard to confine a sick person—especially a child—to their bedroom. As a mom of three,

I know firsthand the challenges of coaxing little bodies to stay put in their rooms. Sick or not, they want to be part of the family. Often, they'll see this as adding insult to injury. They feel miserable, and being sent to their room feels more like punishment. Give it the old college try anyway. The extra cajoling required will reduce exposure to the rest of the family and comes with the side benefit of limiting the number of rooms and surfaces you'll need to tackle, disinfectant in hand, in the days ahead.

Don't Forget the Thermometer

You don't need to go crazy cleaning when a thermometer is repeatedly used on the same person. But before sharing, wipe a thermometer with rubbing alcohol applied to a cotton ball. Rinse well any part that will come near a mouth (not the display), and allow to air-dry thoroughly before using or putting away. The steps are the same whether the model is digital, ear, rectal, or temporal.

To make short work of the latter, strategically position tubs of disinfecting wipes or a disinfectant spray in key locations around the house in a way that encourages use by everyone residing in your home. Some of the stash places you might want to consider: near frequently used surfaces, such as TV remotes, bathroom and kitchen faucet handles and doorknobs, and the home's main light switches— the ones you flick when you come in the door.

While your loved one is sick (and if they're old enough, if the sick one is a child), encourage them to not only use "their" bathroom and bedroom exclusively but to clean the rooms after using them if they feel well enough to do so. If not, well, there goes the daily schedule. If you are the designated cleaner, try not to dash in after each use to tidy up. You should wait as long as possible before entering to clean and disinfect the rooms to give lingering germs and viruses time to clear the air.

SPREAD PROTECTION, NOT GERMS

One of the most important steps is having the sick person stay in designated rooms, away from the other people in the house (as much as possible). More smart steps to help your loved one get back to health and keep everyone else feeling good include the following:

- Use disposable gloves when cleaning areas around the sick person. And only go in a designated sick room to clean when necessary, such as when a wastebasket is overflowing with used tissues—or worse. This will limit your contact with the person who is ill and the germs that landed them that way.

  Wear gloves when there is any contact with the sick person's blood, stool, or other bodily fluids, such as saliva, mucus, vomit, or urine. Throw the used gloves in the lined trash can, and immediately wash your hands when you've finished tidying up.

- Provide your ill family member with a face covering he can wear when you come in to prevent spreading viruses or germs to you.

- If you're sharing a bathroom with your sick family member: ask them to clean and disinfect the surfaces with the disinfecting wipes you've conveniently stashed near the sink if they feel up to it. Other cleaning supplies you might want to have handy include tissues, paper towels, and surface-specific cleaners, such as a toilet bowl cleaner and a bathroom tub and tile cleaner.

- If asking your ill loved one to do this is out of the question, use a face mask to guard against airborne germs, and wait as long as possible after the ill person has last been in the bathroom before coming in to clean or use the restroom yourself.

- If you are sharing space elsewhere, such as a bedroom, let fresh air inside. Open windows or keep doors open during the day to push out as much infected air as possible, so clean air moves through the house, creating a less infectious environment.

- Place a disposable trash bag in the wastebasket. Consider adding a second wastebasket for the sick person's use to keep infectious germs away from you and other healthy bodies in your home. While caring for your loved one and keeping things tidy, avoid touching used tissues and other bedroom waste while emptying wastebaskets. Always wash your hands after emptying wastebaskets, or inadvertently touching used tissues and similar waste, even when wearing gloves.

- To prevent getting sick, avoid touching your eyes, nose, and mouth with unwashed hands; if you can, even avoid it when your hands are clean.

- Remind everyone in the home to regularly wash their hands with soap and water for at least 20 seconds after being near the ill person. Or use a hand sanitizer that contains at least 70 percent alcohol.

SERIOUS SURFACE DISINFECTING

The importance of surface *disinfecting* increases when someone in your household has the telltale signs of a cold or another virus or complains of an upset tummy. Begin cleaning and disinfecting common surfaces and toys in your home as soon as signs of illness pop up and daily until symptoms disappear.

The best defense against infectious diseases is to get serious about surface cleaning. (Combined with frequent handwashing, of course.) By focusing your cleaning efforts on your home's frequently touched objects and surfaces, using the disinfectant cleaner as a weapon of good and shooting to kill the nasty germs in and out of sight, you can win the battle of the bugs (and infectious germs) in your home. And, if you have kids, why not make a game of it? You can triumph over whatever illness has invaded your castle.

When infectious bugs ride into your home on the bottom of your purse or briefcase, or inside your child's backpack, be prepared to greet them, disinfectant in hand. Anytime something taken outside is brought back in, consider it fair game for disinfecting.

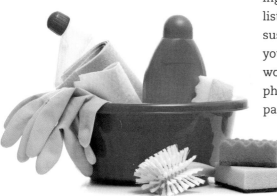

What to put on your target list? The usual frequently touched suspects, naturally: the bottom of your purse, the soles of the shoes worn by everyone inside, and cell phones. While you're at it, take a pass at the less mobile but equally germy high-touch places in your home: light switches, keyboards, remote controls, and doorknobs.

These places are often teeming with many of the more than 200 sneeze- and cough-inducing cold and flu viruses we see today. Without your disinfecting intervention, these annoying interlopers can survive for hours on many hard surfaces in our homes, including plastic and metal surfaces and children's toys.

Hit Surfaces Hard

Cleaning the counters with soapy water can get rid of some germs and make things look tidy—and that may be just fine when everyone in your household is healthy. However, when someone has the flu or a stomach bug, cleaning alone just won't cut it. You want to kill the germs, and water and mild cleaners won't do the trick. When the task at hand requires killing tough viruses and bacteria—not bathing them, it's time to bring in the howitzers of the cleaning world: disinfectants.

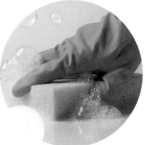

I'm not implying you should ditch cleaning surfaces with soap and water. Surface cleaning removes dirt and grime that, if left intact, provides a significant barrier against the chemical properties of disinfectants, rendering them ineffective. Cleaning is just part one.

When cleaning and disinfecting counters, tabletops, doorknobs, and bed frames, take it one step at a time.

1. Wash the surface with soap and water to first remove dirt and grime and clear the way for the disinfectant's work.

2. Apply your disinfecting cleaner to the surface until visibly wet. Allow it to do its dirty work on the surface for at least 10 minutes. Rinse and wipe dry.

CHOOSING A DISINFECTANT CLEANER

Look for a cleaner with the word *disinfectant* on the label. Ammonia and vinegar, contrary to popular opinion, do not kill bacteria or viruses. For that, you'll need an EPA-certified disinfectant. When using a commercial cleaner, follow the directions for use found on the product label.

If you don't have a commercial disinfectant handy, mix your own with chlorine bleach and laundry detergent:
- ¼ cup bleach
- 1 gallon warm water
- 1 tablespoon powdered laundry detergent.

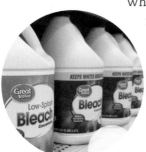

When using a diluted bleach solution, freshness matters. Chlorine bleach loses its chemical cleaning properties when exposed to open air for long time periods. After mixing, a diluted bleach solution should be used within 24 hours to ensure effectiveness.

To disinfect using your homemade bleach solution, dip a paper towel or cotton cloth in the cleaning solution, and apply it to the surface until visibly wet. Let sit for at least 10 minutes. Rinse the surface clean and let dry. For convenience, you can also use the bleach solution in a spray bottle.

According to the CDC, hydrogen peroxide is another safe and effective DIY way to kill bacteria, viruses, and fungi on hard nonporous surfaces. For use as a disinfectant at home, use the 3 percent hydrogen peroxide found at your local grocery store or pharmacy. You can use it right out of the bottle; let sit on the surface for 1 minute before wiping dry.

Rubbing alcohol with 70 percent concentration will kill most bacteria and fungi and many viruses, but it evaporates very quickly. That quick evaporation means it's best used on small and hard surfaces. You'll need to keep the surface visibly wet for a minimum of 30 seconds to ensure the alcohol destroys all germs. It could be helpful for computer keyboards, remote controls, smartphones, and anything else with a touchscreen. Just don't soak your electronics or get liquid near any openings.

CHOOSING YOUR APPLICATION TOOL

When applying and wiping up a cleaning solution, you can use paper towels that can be tossed away after use, machine-washable cotton cloth or rags, or microfiber cloths that can be sanitized in the washing machine after each use. (When drying microfiber cloths, don't use fabric softener sheets; these reduce the woven fibers' effectiveness.)

Then there is that old favorite standby—the sponge. Its ability to soak up spills—and water for rinsing surfaces clean—is its best feature. What would we do without these handy helpers for washing dishes and wiping counters clean? After using your sponge, always rinse it under running water to remove crumbs and dirt from its absorbent surface. If you neglect this step, you'll discover that the sponge's best feature is also its worst. The sponge absorbs and holds everything that isn't a hard surface or nailed down, nasty things like dirt and germs from sinks and counters and errant juice from drippy grocery store meat packages. Without regular disinfecting—the microwave is your best bet here (see page 85 for complete instructions)—bacteria can quickly overrun them.

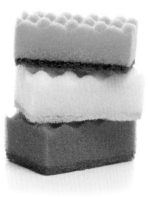

Although I've always been a strong proponent of reducing, reusing, and recycling, there are times when using disposable wipes and paper towels is a safer and more convenient choice. Cleaning the toilet and mopping up pet accidents are two examples. Containing a confirmed sickness in the household is another key time. Wipe away the mess and toss, eliminating the chance for germs to spread.

GEAR UP FOR SAFE CLEANING

Start every cleaning session with gloves—disposable rubber, vinyl, or latex—to keep germs from taking a ride on your hands and spreading to any and every surface you touch. They also

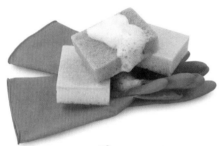

protect your skin against harsh cleaning products, such as bleach, that can irritate or burn the skin. Toss them or wash them when you're done (depending on the type). Always wash your hands thoroughly after a cleaning session, even one when you're wearing gloves. Don't skip this step.

If you use a sponge or washable cleaning cloth, designate one for use in each room to prevent spreading germs between rooms, such as between the bathroom and kitchen. Use different colors in each room to help keep them straight.

ROOM-BY-ROOM GUIDE

To stay on top of germs during cold and flu seasons or when someone in your home is sick, regularly disinfect high-touch surfaces or those that the ill person has touched. Give special attention to surfaces in the ill person's bedroom and bathroom. Critical surfaces to hit include bedside tables, countertops, sinks and faucet handles, remote controls and computer keyboards, doorknobs, light switches, tub or shower, and toilets (including the entire seat and the toilet handle).

While the illness is running its course, you'll want to take the following room-by-room precautions to keep everyone in your home healthy and bug- or virus-free.

Keep the Kitchen Safe

Pay close cleaning attention to the kitchen and its various surfaces. The kitchen is the room in which people tend to gather and touch things, and it is where food and drinks are prepared and often served. Bacteria and viruses can live on the surfaces here for days, even weeks.

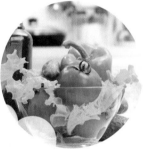

BE A CAREFUL COOK. To prevent spreading germs to the rest of the household, the sick person should not be the one who prepares meals for the rest of the family. Even the most meticulous hand-washing may not be enough to keep everyone safe, especially from easily spread germs causing illnesses like the norovirus.

Stomach bug–causing viruses like unpleasant rotavirus can easily wiggle their way into food and meal prep areas, given the slightest opportunity, and spread quickly through hand-to-mouth contact. If you're the one who's sick, for your family's safety, don't prepare meals or other food until you have been symptom-free for at least 48 hours. Whoever does the food prep and cooking should disinfect everything touched, such as the refrigerator, microwave, other appliances, drawer handles, faucets, and stove knobs.

GIVE DISHES DUE DILIGENCE. You should avoid sharing knives, forks, spoons, and dishes used by a sick person in your home. Please don't use these items until you have washed them, either in the dishwasher or by hand in warm soapy water, and dried thoroughly. Moisture anywhere provides the ideal environment for pathogens to grow and multiply.

Wash all utensils and dishes used by the infected family members at high heat in the dishwasher. Treat them to a disinfectant cleaning solution (e.g., 4 teaspoons of bleach per gallon of warm water) if hand-washing; rinse thoroughly.

When Sharing Isn't Caring

In addition to dishes and utensils, do not share or allow anyone in your home to share or use towels, bedding, or electronics (like a cell phone or game controller) that have recently been used or handled by the ill family member.

If you are healthy and wish to remain that way, protect yourself by wearing gloves when handling or washing dishes and utensils used by your ill family member. Even when using gloves to bus and wash dishes and utensils, you should still wash your hands with soap and water after taking the gloves off.

PATROL SURFACES WITH DISINFECTANT. The kitchen surface patrol includes tables, chair backs, refrigerator handles, the sink, countertops, drawers, and cabinet hardware. Clean and wipe daily with disinfectant wipes or disinfectant spray.

DINE WITH SOCIAL DISTANCE. Serve your ill family member meals in their bedroom or a separate area of your home. A patio area works, too. Putting some distance between the sickie and the rest of the household will limit airborne germs between family members. Once again, you're likely to meet some resistance. Toe the line as much as possible here. Your health and that of the others in your home—big and small—depend on keeping the risk of transmission low.

Bust Bedroom Germs

When you're sick, your bed is usually the go-to spot for some much-needed rest. But all that time spent horizontal with a bad cold or virus gives germs and bacteria plenty of time to get comfy too.

KICK GERMS OUT OF BED. It's essential to sanitize the bed linens in the warmest water possible and dry thoroughly when the worst has passed. If you can't avoid sharing a bedroom with the sick person, sanitizing is especially important. Change the pillow-case that your sick partner has coughed or sneezed on daily, and you might fare better. No need to change the other bed linens unless they get soiled. If you're dealing with diarrhea or vomiting (see Sick Stain Busters, page 157), wash clothes, soiled linens, or stuffed toys right away. Don't shake them to fluff or for any other reason. You're trying to avoid spreading germs, remember?

FOCUS ON HIGH-TOUCH SPOTS. Clean and disinfect objects the sick person has come into contact with on an as-needed basis. For example, if a sick person is only moving from the bed to the bath-room and back, pay close cleaning attention to the nightstand, the bathroom door handle, bedposts, changing tables, and anything else front and center that could potentially be germy. Pacifiers and toys with hard surfaces without batteries or attached parts can go in the dishwasher.

TACKLE THE TRASH. Use a lined wastebasket in the sick person's room to minimize contact between you and the germy contents inside when taking out the trash. Empty the sick room waste-basket bin at least once daily, replacing the bag each time with a fresh one.

Expect the wastebasket to get pretty disgusting—especially if the sick person vomits into it. To disinfect the wastebasket, remove the liner bag and rinse well. Then wipe the inside and outside of the wastebasket with a solution of ½ cup of bleach and ¾ gallon of water. Let the solution sit disinfecting for 10 minutes, then rinse and allow it to air-dry.

Clean after the All Clear

Once an illness has run its course, clean and disinfect the room (or rooms) that the sick person used and any items inside they may have touched. Throw away and replace the ill person's toothbrush; clean and disinfect the toothbrush holder and grooming tools with warm soapy water or put them in the dishwasher (if dishwasher safe).

CLEAR THE AIR. Dust can be extra irritating when someone is sick. Dust furniture around the room they are staying in, especially the headboard and the nightstand, and vacuum the floor every few days or more often if needed. Don't forget the corners and under the bed.

If weather allows, open the windows to give stagnant germ-filled air a way out and to usher fresh air in. They don't need to stay open all day, just long enough to bring fresh air in and move infected air out.

Battle the Bathroom

Bathrooms are home to plenty of germy problem areas that only get germier and more problematic when someone is sick. Give everything you encounter in here a serious sanitizing.

CALL IN THE DISINFECTANT. Use a disinfectant cleaner on tooth-paste tubes and toiletries handled by the sick person; the trash can; doorknobs; light switches; sink and shower handles; the toilet seat, lid, and handle; and the area on the floor around the toilet.

GUARD TOOTHBRUSHES. While you're there, clean everyone's toothbrushes with soap and water or in the dishwasher. Alternatively, you could just replace them. You should be replacing them roughly every six months, anyway. If it's about that time, make that move.

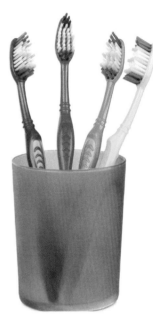

If family members share a toothbrush holder, it is imperative to separate the infected person's toothbrushes from the toothbrushes of others in the home who are not yet infected, so germs do not spread from one toothbrush to another due to proximity. Use disposable rinsing cups.

SEPARATE TOWELS. Designate a hand towel to be used only by the ill person or change hand towels daily. You can also switch to paper towels during the illness to prevent the inadvertent use of a shared towel that could result in the transfer of germs to others in your home.

Clean Those Living Spaces

The family room and living room are popular gathering spots in many homes. And, where we go, our germs go, too. We sit on the sofa, chill in chairs, channel search on the carpet, with all these surfaces collecting viruses and bacteria in the process.

COVER THE RISK. Keep contamination of upholstered furniture and accessories in these rooms to a minimum by covering these items and areas with washable sheets or blankets. Wash and change the protective throws frequently. Remove any decorative pillows or cover them with washable pillowcases.

MAP OUT A FOCUS. Think about where the sick person rested and plan your room chores accordingly. Airborne viruses travel up to three feet when someone coughs or sneezes. If your little one is sick, think about where he puts his mouth and his curious hands, and clean those areas, too. Board games or gaming controllers handled by the ill family member should always be cleaned and sanitized before anyone else in the home uses them.

HIT HIGH-TOUCH SURFACES. Don't forget to disinfect all the room's high-touch surfaces, including the television remote, phones, computer keyboards, and door-knobs leading in and out and to other rooms. For steps to sanitize sensitive electronics, see page 89.

HANDLING GERMY LAUNDRY SAFELY

Making a clean bed can bring some much-needed comfort when someone is feeling sick. While you want to keep the ill person comfy to expedite their recovery process, you also want to prevent yourself and other family members from becoming sick. The ideal way to do this is by combining safe laundry handling habits with laundry additives and laundry disinfectants.

When you're taking care of any sick persons in your home, take extra care with laundry.

Glove Up
One of the smartest things that you can do to protect yourself from catching something is to wear disposable or reusable gloves when handling soiled laundry. Wash your hands thoroughly afterward.

Be a Speedy Germ Remover
Immediately remove and wash clothes or bedding that has blood, stool, or bodily fluids on them to prevent cross-contamination. Give the sick person a separate hamper or washable laundry bag to contain these items.

Keep It Still and Distanced
A sick person's towels, bedding, and clothes are full of germs, so don't "hug" their dirty clothes while transporting or sorting. You should never shake out the dirty laundry of someone who is ill, as this can project their germs into the air and your respiratory system or onto other surfaces. To avoid spreading viruses and bacteria, touch dirty laundry as little as possible. Instead, carry dirty clothes in a laundry basket or a washable or disposable bag and dump right into the washing machine when you're ready.

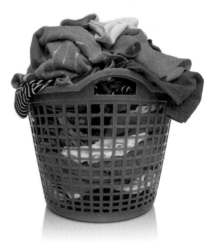

Know When to Separate
Doing the sick person's laundry doesn't have to mean extra work on wash day. Unless bodily fluids have sullied the collected

clothes or linens, you can wash the sick person's dirty laundry with everyone else's dirty duds. There's no need to set the items aside for a solo wash or wait to run a load.

Become a Voracious Label Reader

Washing clothes in the warmest water safe for the fabric is not only an essential step in sanitizing an ill person's laundry; it's a best practice for getting all your wash day loads clean. Get in the habit of reading a garment's care label before tossing it in the machine, especially the first time you wash it. Warmer water helps laundry detergent more effectively loosen up and remove stains and body oils, so they can 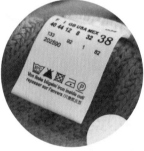 be washed away in the rinse water. If the care label designates, dry the ill person's laundry on medium to high heat. Laundering items in the hottest water safe for the fabric, combined with heated drying for at least 45 minutes, is an essential part of the sanitizing process. (See Chapter 6, starting on page 125, for more on disinfecting laundry.)

Don't Forget Containers

Clean and disinfect laundry hampers and baskets after use. If possible, use separate clothes hampers and baskets for clean and dirty laundry. Even when using different containers, always clean the interior with a disinfecting wipe or spray after use.

Finish with Your Machine

You should always disinfect your washing machine after cleaning and washing the bedsheets, clothes, and towels of an infected person in your home to prevent the spread of germs or bacteria to subsequent loads. The washer's moist environment is a breeding ground for germs. Disinfecting the machine is especially crucial if you mainly use cold water for washing as hot water kills the bacteria both on clothes and in the machine. (See page 120 for info on how to disinfect a washer and dryer.)

SICK STAIN BUSTERS

Because accidents happen, especially when we don't feel well, here's how to remove stains like vomit, urine, spilled liquid medicines, and blood.

Blood

Rinse and presoak the soiled garment in cold water, then machine wash in cold water. Do not add chlorine bleach or use warm water for washing, as bleach and heat can cause a protein-based stain to set.

Feces

Combine 1 teaspoon of liquid dishwashing detergent and 2 cups of cold water. Dip a cloth or sponge in the enzyme laundry detergent solution, and blot on the stained area, moving the cloth around and rewetting as needed until the stain lightens or disappears. Launder in the warmest water the fabric can handle with bleach or other laundry sanitizers safe for the fabric. (See page 133 for more on laundry sanitizers.)

Liquid Medicines

Rinse under warm, running water to help loosen up the gunk for removal. This step is especially important if the mixture has dried on the item. Use a cloth to blot an

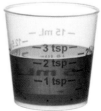

enzyme laundry detergent solution (1 teaspoon of liquid dishwashing detergent in 2 cups of cold water) on the stained area until damp but not soaking wet. Let sit on the fabric for several minutes, then rinse thoroughly.

Repeat these steps as needed until you have removed as much of the stain's visible color as possible. If the stain remains, soak the area in cold water for at least 30 minutes, occasionally agitating the fabric with your fingers. Launder using the warmest water safe for the fabric.

Urine

Rinse the soiled area with cold water, then soak overnight in an enzyme laundry detergent solution (1 teaspoon of liquid dishwashing detergent in 2 cups of cold water). Machine wash in the warmest water that is safe for the fabric with a laundry sanitizer.

Vomit

Scrape any solids off the garment. (I didn't say this would be pleasant work.) Dampen the discolored area with water, then sprinkle with baking soda until the stain is covered. (The baking soda will absorb the smell and help loosen the stain from the fabric's fibers.) Lightly moisten the area with lemon juice or vinegar. (It will fizz.) Using a toothbrush or your fingers, gently rub the goop into the fabric to remove as much of the stain as possible. Rinse the solution from the fabric under running water. Machine wash as usual.

When your household is healthy, you'll all be back on the go. As you head beyond your home or invite deliveries in, some powerful steps in Chapter 8 can offer protection against germs because they don't take days off.

HOMEMADE STAIN SOLUTIONS

Try these homemade stain busters the next time you need to remove a clothing blight:

Household ammonia mix
Add 1 part ammonia to 8 parts water.

Enzyme detergent mix
Add 1 teaspoon of laundry detergent to 1 cup of water.

Hand-dishwashing liquid mix
Add 1 teaspoon of liquid dishwashing soap to 1 cup of water.

Hydrogen peroxide
Use 3 percent, undiluted.

Fels-Naptha paste
Shave slices off a Fels-Naptha bar soap. Add 1 part shavings to 10 parts water. Work into a paste.

WD-40
Use full strength.

After treating stains, always wash clothes in the hottest water safe for the fabric, using chlorine bleach or color-safe bleach per the item's care label.

8

GROCERIES, TAKEOUT, PACKAGES & MORE

On-the-Go & Into-Your-Home Precautions

CLEAN FREAK OR NOT, living through a pandemic has probably upped your cleaning game a few levels. Gone are the spray-and-wipe cleaning sprints of yesteryear. You're a super-sanitizer now, taking extra time on high-touch objects and surfaces—like kitchen counters, light switches, and doorknobs—to obliterate the pathogens that could make your family ill.

But new attention is not limited to what you clean around the house. You're likely looking at your surroundings wherever you go a little differently, too. You're learning to be smart about touching common surfaces like door handles, grocery store shopping carts, and restaurant menus outside your home.

You might find yourself in various scenarios while out and about—taking rideshare to work, dining out, or staying in a hotel—that will naturally have you wondering how to prevent the transmission of germs and viruses to remain healthy. You don't need to be a germaphobe during a pandemic to be concerned about your surroundings' cleanliness.

Your new efforts will make sense and can go a long way to keeping your on-the-go family healthy. Pathogenic germs aren't static. They can hitch a ride on you or the many things you carry home with you—your shoes, debit card, even your grocery bags. No, that does not mean a biohazard-level scrubbing should be undertaken on these items upon return. Here's how to protect yourself in a variety of on-the-go situations.

WHEREVER YOU GO

Keeping our hands clean is one of the most important steps we can take to avoid getting sick and spreading germs to others. Although the process isn't rocket science, the CDC and other health experts recommend cleaning hands in a specific way. Whether you're turning to good old-fashioned handwashing with soap and water or applying hand sanitizer, the recommended steps aren't arbitrary; they're based on data and support from a number of studies.

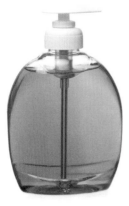

Before the pandemic, you probably didn't think twice about whether you were washing your hands correctly. After all, it's second nature—you've been doing it routinely for years, right? But research has found that as many as 95 percent of us are doing it wrong. Where are we messing up? In a study based on observations of 3,749 people in public restrooms, researchers found that . . .

- Ten percent didn't wash their hands at all.

- Thirty-three percent didn't use soap.

- Ninety-five percent didn't wash long enough to kill the germs that can cause infections. It takes 15 to 20 seconds of vigorous handwashing with soap and water to effectively kill the germs, yet the study found that people are only washing their hands, on average, for about 6 seconds.

- People were less likely to wash their hands if the sink was dirty.

- Handwashing was more prevalent earlier in the day.

- People were more likely to wash their hands if a sign encouraging them to do so was present.

The Right Way to Wash Hands

So, how can we do better?

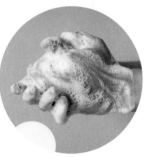

1. WET YOUR HANDS. Use clean running water—warm or cold. The water temperature is a matter of preference and doesn't affect how clean your hands get. No need to scald yourself here.

2. LATHER UP. Apply a quarter-sized amount of soap. Using soap to wash hands is more effective than using water alone because the surfactants in soap lift soil and microbes from the skin, and people tend to scrub hands more thoroughly when using soap, which further removes germs.

3. SCRUB FOR 20 SECONDS. Rub your hands together to create a good lather, and scrub under your nails, between your fingers, and the backs of your hands. The friction helps lift

dirt, grease, and microbes from the skin. You should wash for at least 20 seconds—humming the "Happy Birthday" song from start to end twice is one way to track the time.

4. RINSE. Rinse your hands well under running water. You'll be sending all the germs you lifted off your hands down the drain.

5. AVOID RECONTAMINATION. When finished, turn off the faucet with a paper towel, then dry your hands using a clean towel or air-dry them. Germs can be transferred more easily to and from wet hands, so don't skip this step.

When using a public restroom, after washing your hands, make sure not to touch any surfaces on your way out the door, which you should plan to use a clean paper towel to open.

Using Hand Sanitizer Is Simple

Washing hands with soap and water is the best way to get rid of germs in most situations. Soap and water not readily available, or facing a sink that's downright frightening? As long as it contains at least 60 percent alcohol, hand sanitizer is a smart alternative to traditional handwashing. You can tell if the sanitizer contains at least 60 percent alcohol by looking at the product label.

- Use one or two squirts or pumps of the product.

- Rub hands together briskly, including the front and back, between fingers, and around and under nails, until hands are dry.

Caution with Kids

Swallowing alcohol-based hand sanitizer can cause alcohol poisoning if more than a couple of mouthfuls are swallowed. Keep it out of reach of young children and supervise their use.

Sanitizers can quickly reduce the number of germs on hands in many situations. However . . .

- Sanitizers do not get rid of all types of germs.

- Hand sanitizers may not be as effective when hands are visibly dirty or greasy.

- Hand sanitizers might not remove harmful chemicals from hands like pesticides and heavy metals.

TAKE CARE IN YOUR CAR

Just like we regularly clean and disinfect frequently touched surfaces in our homes, we should do the same in our cars. Give attention to the steering wheel, gear shift, doorframes and handles, windows and window controls, radio and temperature dials, and seatbelt buckles. This sanitizing is even more important if multiple members of a household use the car.

Stay Stocked for Safety

Keep disinfecting wipes in the car for easy touch-ups, and you'll have peace of mind knowing that the number of mobile germs will be limited. High-touch surfaces in our vehicles can hold virus-carrying particles that can be transmitted from our hands to our eyes, nose, or mouth.

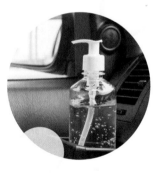

Park Those Germs

Consider using alcohol wipes on parking meters and pay stations to disinfect the surfaces before inserting your card or cash. After taking care of business, use a hand sanitizer containing at least 60 percent alcohol. Then wash your hands with soap and water for at least 20 seconds as soon as it is possible.

SANITIZE YOUR SHADES

For most of us, our sunglasses are always on board when we hit the road. Our stylish specs do more than just protect our eyes from the sun, however. They also serve as a significant barrier between us and the respiratory droplets of a coughing or sneezing passenger or stranger.

Viruses can live on glass for up to four days, and for up to the three days on plastic and stainless steel materials used in lenses and frames. Make sure to clean them regularly with soap and water:

- Rinse the lenses of your sunglasses with water first to avoid scratching the surface of the lenses.
- Place a drop or two of dish soap onto the lens, and swirl it around gently with a microfiber cloth. You can also use disposable lens cleaner wipes, made specifically for this purpose.
- Clean the nose pads and the edge where the lens and frame intersect. These touch the face repeatedly and can become very dirty.
- Clean the frame of the glasses, as well as the earpieces that go behind the ears.
- Rinse and dry with a soft lint-free cloth. Don't use paper towels, which contain fibers that can easily scratch the lenses. If using non-disposable material to clean your glasses, be sure to wash that cloth after cleaning your sunglasses.

Worried about possibly rusting the screws in your frame? The risk of rusting is low, and even so, those little screws are easily replaceable.

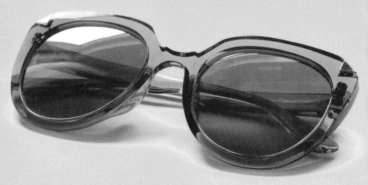

Fuel Clean Habits

When getting gas, wipe the nozzle handle and screen buttons with a disinfecting wipe. After fueling, use a 60 percent alcohol hand sanitizer. Wash your hands for at least 20 seconds with soap and water when you get home or arrive at the next pit stop.

Welcome Fresh Air

If you can, improve your car's ventilation simply by opening windows or setting the air ventilation or air-conditioning on non-recirculation mode.

Choose Passengers Carefully

Limit how many passengers are allowed in your car. While it's never fun to whittle down the group, it's best to stick with healthy family members rather than half the neighborhood.

PROTECTION ON PUBLIC TRANSPORTATION

If you regularly take the bus or subway, you are six times more likely to get sick than if you'd hoofed it or driven yourself. Why? Easy. The more people you come into contact with, the more germs you are exposed to. If a train or bus looks overcrowded, it may pay to wait for the next one.

When using any type of transportation, the CDC recommends following these general principles:

- Upon arrival, wash your hands with soap and water for at least 20 seconds, or sanitize your hands with a 60 percent alcohol solution.

- Don't touch your eyes, nose, or mouth if your hands are unwashed.

- Cover your cough and sneezes with a tissue or use the inside of your elbow. Throw used tissues in the trash (keep the elbow) and wash your hands immediately with soap and water or use hand sanitizer.

- Avoid frequently touched surfaces, such as kiosks, touch-screens, ticket machines, turnstiles, elevator buttons, handrails, restroom surfaces, and public benches as much as possible. Wash your hands with soap and water, or use a hand sanitizer as soon as possible if you touch one of these surfaces.

- When available, choose touchless payment. Use no-touch trash cans and doors when you can. Place any payment required in a tray or on a counter instead of handing it directly to an agent.

VIGILANCE WITH SHARED VEHICLES

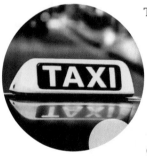

To stay safe and reduce exposure to germs when using a shared ride service (like Uber or Lyft), taxi, limo, or for-hire vehicle:

- Avoid contact with frequently touched surfaces, such as the car's doorframes, handles, and windows. When such contact is unavoidable, use a hand sanitizer containing at least 60 percent alcohol as soon as possible afterward.

- Avoid accepting water bottles and touching magazines or other items provided for free to passengers.

- Use touchless payment when available.

- Opt out of pools or rides in which drivers make frequent stops to pick up multiple passengers.

- When riding in larger vehicles like buses or vans, choose a seat in the back so you are at least six feet from the driver.

- Ask the driver to improve the vehicle's ventilation by opening the windows or setting the air ventilation or air-conditioning on non-recirculation mode.

- After leaving the vehicle, apply a 60 percent alcohol-containing hand sanitizer.

- Wash your hands in soap and water for at least 20 seconds when you reach your destination.

When using or riding shared bikes, scooters, skateboards, and other micro-mobility devices, follow the general principles listed above for safety's sake. Additionally, before you hop on or skate off into the sunset, take a disinfecting wipe to frequently touched surfaces, such as handlebars, gears, brake handles, and locks.

SAFER PLANES AND TRAINS

Whenever you have lots of people in a tight space with limited airflow for a few hours, germ buildup is inevitable. Still, you can take some simple steps to lower your exposure.

Skip Seat Pockets

Studies have shown that seat pockets are some of the worst offenders when it comes to germs. Why? You know this one. It's because we use seat pockets as a trash bin more often than as a storage space. Passengers have been known to stuff everything from dirty diapers to used tissues in those germy seat pockets.

SANITIZING SURPRISE
Silver Is Valuable against Germs

The bacteria-killing properties of silver have been known for centuries, although it is still a mystery as to exactly how the metal works this antimicrobial magic. You can find tiny silver particles in specially designed cutting boards, yoga mats, and apparel—especially underwear, socks, and bags.

Researchers at Auburn University found MRSA could survive in seat pocket material for up to 168 hours—more than enough time for many passengers to contract this nasty infection. So, the next time you need to stash something, skip the seat pocket. It's just not worth the risk. Instead, stow your stuff in a protective carry-on bag with silver-ion technology that destroys germs.

Bypass the Bin

You probably shouldn't reach for the overhead bin to store your stuff, either. The overhead bin latches get a lot of handling, especially during the boarding process, and little to no cleaning, according to a *USA Today* report. As passengers walk down the aisle, repeatedly opening and closing bins in search of a spot to stash their coat or bag, latches on the bins become fertile ground for growing bacteria, viruses, and other microbes.

So walk on by the overhead bins. Instead, slide your carry-on under the seat in front of you. In addition to being convenient, it's surprisingly cleaner.

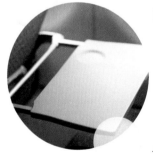

Stay Away from Trays

You'll want to take a disinfectant wipe to the tray table before you set your drink—or anything else—on it. Travelmath's researchers found that tray tables have an astounding 2,155 colony-forming units per square inch. As if that weren't scary enough, researchers at Auburn University found these hardy bacteria can survive on the plastic surface for up to three days. Even after you've used a disinfectant wipe on the surface, you'd be better off avoiding as much contact as possible. Sanitize your hands immediately after any tray use.

Stick to Your Own Touchscreens

It's going to be a long flight. Good thing you have hundreds of movies, games, and music options to choose from on the entertainment system in front of you. Or is it? Chances are, virtually everyone who occupied that seat before you had their hands on that touchscreen. Instead of risking the germs that may be lurking, bring your own entertainment—a book, laptop, or smartphone. But if you still want to watch a movie, break out the hand sanitizer. Avoid touching your face after using the screen to keep germs and bacteria in their place (not yours).

ENJOY A SANITIZED HOTEL STAY

Worried about a hotel stop? Keep things safe throughout your travels by choosing online options for check-in (and checkout) and contactless payment. Another smart step: always carry a tub of disinfecting wipes in your carry-on.

Most hotel chains have put stringent cleaning protocols in place for in-room surfaces and clean public areas frequently. Still, clean freaks would probably feel more at home giving the room's surfaces a quick once-over with a disinfecting wipe before settling in.

The germiest spots in hotel rooms? The bathroom counter and faucet, the desk, and—just like at home—light switches and remote controls. Don't let this news have you swearing off travel forever. These dirty issues can be cleaned up (mostly), too.

CLEAN CHOICES
Be Picky with Pillows

Hotel pillows . . . need I say more? If you're concerned about potential allergens and bacteria, throw a travel pillow in your bag and avoid using the hotel pillow altogether. Another option: bring along your own zip-up case to slide that pillow inside.

Face the Counter and Faucet

To quell your quivering inner germaphobe, wipe down your faucets and counters with disinfecting wipes before using and before placing your items on the surface.

Deal with Desks

You'd be well served giving the desk in your hotel room a thorough cleaning once (or twice) with disinfecting wipes before setting your bag, laptop, and business documents on it. Respiratory viruses can live on the surface for up to four days.

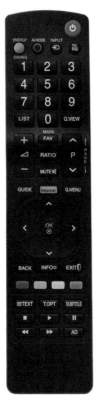

Sanitize Light Switches

According to a University of Houston study, the first thing we usually touch upon entering a hotel room is the light switch, which happens to be the hotel room's dirtiest surface. The study found that the main light switches often contained high levels of fecal bacteria. Don't let this unpleasant life truth ruffle your feathers. Now that you know, just be prepared with a disinfecting wipe in hand upon entering your hotel room; use it to flip or turn on the light switch and wipe clean the surface.

Clean Remote Controls

Just like at home, the TV remotes in hotel rooms are germ cesspools. Studies have found that remote controls are one of the germiest things in most hotel rooms. An easy fix: just grab the ice bucket plastic liner or hotel shower cap and use it to cover the remote control, so you're able to turn the TV on and off and change channels without getting bugged.

BEAT GERMS AT THE GYM

It's a lot to take in. Planes, trains, and automobiles . . . and now even the cozy hotel room you'd been looking forward to unwinding in is presenting challenges to your health, too. You need to blow off some steam. Time to hit the gym!

A serious sweat sesh might be just what the doctor ordered to help relieve stress and keep you healthy. Good idea (mostly). It turns out fitness junkies have some nasty habits. According to a survey of 2,000 people conducted by Nuffield Health, a UK health firm, 74 percent said fellow gym-goers didn't wipe down sweaty equipment; 49 percent used water bottles, towels, and toiletries that weren't theirs; 18 percent went to the gym sick; and 16 percent didn't wash their gym clothes between workouts. That said, there's no need to scrap the workout plan altogether.

Gyms can be gross, sure, but there's no scientific evidence that gyms will make you sick. For a cleaner workout session, continue doing what you already do (i.e., wiping down surfaces you frequently touch) and practice good gym hygiene. These simple steps will limit your exposure to gym germs that cause cold, flu, norovirus, athlete's foot, and staph infections.

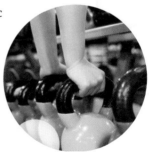

Wipe, Wash, Wipe

Keeping your hands clean with hand sanitizer and wiping down each machine or set of weights before and after you use it with disinfectant wipes provided by your gym will help keep germs at bay.

Shower Smarter

When it's time to hit the showers, don't go barefoot. Although they're not foolproof, wearing slip-resistant flip-flops in the shower will provide a barrier between you and the floors. Pop the flops in a plastic bag after you've cleaned up your act.

Fungal spores can still get on your shower shoes, however. To minimize the risk, soak your shower shoes in a diluted bleach solution once in a while. That safeguard will help keep them and your feet as clean and fungus-free as possible.

Clean Your Gym Wear

Dark moist gym bags are an ideal growing ground for fungi. To keep your gym bag clean, put your dirty duds in a plastic bag. And, don't forget your workout shoes. Slip them in a plastic bag too before tossing them into your gym bag. When you get home, wipe them clean (including the bottoms) with a disinfecting wipe. Allow to air-dry.

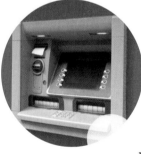

CLEANING UP AT THE ATM

At some point, while you're out and about, you'll inevitably need to replenish the cash supply. Simple, right? Staying germ-free during the transaction? Not so much. Chances are, you aren't the first person to use the ATM today. This means you could be picking up germs and who knows what else left behind from every person who completed a transaction at the machine today.

Your best defense is a good offense, in the form of a quick pre-transaction surface wipe-down with a disinfecting wipe. If your bank doesn't offer those at its ATMs, use the handy travel pack in your bag (you remembered to pop that in before you left home, right?) to clean things up before you take care of business.

And, the money you take out of the ATM is part of the problem, too. That money is—as our mothers told us many times—dirty. Researchers have found that most dollar bills are home to more than 3,000 types of microorganisms. So, have that hand sanitizer ready as soon as you stash the cash away.

Even the card you put in the machine to get that cash can be part of the problem. You might think money is the dirtiest item in your wallet, but our debit and credit cards may be home to far more microbes than our cold cash. It all depends on us— how often we use it and where it's been.

Not a problem, though; this plastic can be cleaned up quickly with items you probably already have at home, underneath the sink. To clean, use a disinfecting wipe or a disinfectant cleaner sprayed on a cotton ball or paper towel. Gently wipe both sides of the card with the cleaner and allow it to air-dry before putting it back into action.

Safe for Chips and Strips?

Your plastic credit cards are water-resistant, which means you can clean the card's chip and magnetic strip the same way you clean the rest of your card. Your cards are sturdy but not indestructible, so don't give your cards too vigorous a scrubbing. A gentle hand is best. Make sure your card's magnetic strip and chip are completely dry before you slip it back in your wallet.

If you don't have a disinfectant cleaner or disinfecting wipe, wash the card in warm water and a squirt or two of dishwashing soap. Be sure to clean both sides. If grime has attached itself to any card numbers, use a toothpick to get it out. Rinse and allow to air-dry.

NAVIGATING GROCERY STORES

You don't need to wipe down every package you bring home, but a few smart steps can go a long way to avoiding or killing germs you may pick up along with dinner.

Beware the Cart Cesspool

Meat juices in the basket. Overflowing diapers in the seat. Bomber birds in the parking lot. No wonder shopping cart handles and seats are home to severe nasties like *Salmonella*, *E. coli*, and *Campylobacter*. Before you race off down the aisles in your frantic search for dinner, make a safety pit stop at the disinfecting wipes dispenser (if your store provides one). Cover all the places your hands might wander during the dinner race.

Keep a Circle of Space

Once inside, the most significant risk to your health comes from your fellow shoppers. To limit contact, shop during hours when fewer people will be there (e.g., early mornings or late at night), and try to stay six feet away from everyone else, just to be safe.

Check Out with Care

Choose touchless payment (i.e., paying without touching money, a card, or a keypad) if possible. If you must handle money or a credit card, or use a store keypad, sanitize your hands after paying.

Create Safe Returns

Set your grocery bags on the floor of your kitchen instead of the counter to prevent cross-contamination. After unloading the groceries, clean, recycle, or ditch the germy grocery bags and then wash your hands or use a hand sanitizer.

HOW TO WASH REUSABLE BAGS

Studies have shown that most shoppers with reusable bags rarely, if ever, send them for a spin in the washing machine. If you're among them, it's time to come clean. Clean shopping bags can protect you and your foodstuff from all manner of bacterial unpleasantries.

First, clean the insert with a disinfectant wipe or cleaner. Then turn the bag inside out for washing.

- Some natural canvas shopping bags come with care instructions, which always makes life easier. If not, these bags are sturdy enough to machine wash in hot water with laundry detergent. Air-dry if you don't want them to shrink on you.

- Mesh, hand-knit, and crocheted bags need a gentler hand-washing, also in hot water; air-dry.

- If you go the hand-washing route, give the nooks and crannies around the stitched seams a little extra cleaning attention.

- Hand-wash or use your machine's gentle cycle to clean woven plastic (polypropylene) bags. If grocery day didn't coincide with wash day this week, wipe the interior and exterior clean with a disinfecting wipe or spray. Always air-dry—polypropylene bags could melt in the dryer.

- Nylon bags (without insulation) can be washed by hand or machine in warm water, using the gentle cycle. Always air-dry nylon bags. Like their plastic cousins, nylon bags can melt if sent for a tumble in the dryer.

- Insulated shopping bags or totes are easy care embodied. Go over the interior and exterior surfaces with a disinfectant cleaner or wipe after each use.

Or, consider getting some canvas bags you can bring to the grocery store, wash when you get home, and reuse next time. If you don't have time to wash the bags after unloading them, spray the outside of your bags with a disinfectant.

- Do not place clean reusable shopping bags in the germy baby seat and carrier section of your grocery cart.

- Do not use reusable grocery bags to tote around any other items, such as diapers, gym clothes, or beach gear.

- Don't leave unwashed bags in a hot car, where bacteria can thrive and multiply.

SMART DINING AND DELIVERY

Most restaurants have created ever-evolving cleaning protocols to keep you safe, such as setting fewer tables to increase the distance between people, wrapping dining utensils in napkins, and disinfecting surfaces between customers. Menus are a thing of the past at some restaurants, replaced by QR codes, enabling you to peruse the daily specials on your smartphone.

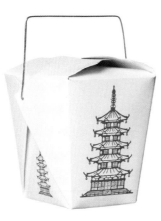

In restaurants that still offer diners a physical menu, if you touch a menu that is not single-use, wash your hands after ordering. If you have a choice in where to sit, choose an outside table.

Skip the communal bread basket to avoid potentially tracking germs from your hand to your mouth. Skipping shared plates and meals, too, is best (sorry). If you're eating family-style, assign one person to serve the table to minimize the number of people touching the serving utensils.

- Stay away from self-serve food and drink options.

- Wash your hands for at least 20 seconds when entering and exiting the restaurant. If you can't get to a sink to wash your hands with soap and water, use a hand sanitizer. Ensure you cover all surfaces of your hands with the sanitizer, then rub your hands together until dry.

Prefer food takeout or delivery to dining in? There's no proven reason to worry about having a delivery person drop off food or supplies. It's a safe and convenient option. However, after handling a delivery and always before eating, it's a good idea to wash your hands with soap and water or use an alcohol-based gel hand sanitizer.

Package Protection

Mail and packages are pretty low risk when it comes to pathogenic germs. The time it took to arrive on your doorstep was likely long enough to inactivate any surface viruses. But it never hurts to open the package, recycle or toss the box, and immediately wash or sanitize your hands. If the delivery comes from a grocery store, spray the outside of reusable bags with a disinfectant, for safety's sake.

It's unlikely that you'd get a virus from touching carryout containers, but it can't hurt to take smart precautions. (We're talking about your health and safety here!) When you get the food container home, empty the contents on to a plate, and toss or recycle the container it came in.

- Choose touchless payment or pay online or on the phone when you order (if possible).

- Accept deliveries without in-person contact whenever possible. To cut down on face-to-face interaction, request that your order be left in a safe spot on your front porch (or lobby).

- After receiving a delivery or bringing home takeout, wash your hands with soap and water or use a 60 percent alcohol hand sanitizer.

GERMS AT WORK

Germs thrive on the surfaces in your workplace as much as the surfaces in your home. If Susie in accounting came down with a doozy of a cold yesterday, you're probably wondering just how long viruses and germs can live on workplace surfaces. The influenza virus can survive on surfaces and still infect you for up to 8 hours after being deposited via sneezing Susie on the copy machine.

Cleaning Doesn't Replace Washing

Remember the little infectors are always on the go and can travel on your hands, moving to and from surfaces throughout the office as you touch them. That's why frequent handwashing is key to stopping the spread of infections.

It's essential to keep all your work surfaces clean, especially your desktop. Additional office items that need regular cleaning attention include computers, telephones, and other electronic equipment. Sensitive expensive electronic office equipment requires unique cleaning methods—see page 89.

Honestly, it's best to avoid shared office food. But if you do share, it can help to outfit the break room, kitchen, or lunch table with sanitizing hand wipes and bakery tissue. If they're within easy reach, chances are most of your coworkers will remember to wipe down their hands before picking up a bakery tissue to grab a donut from the box.

Be cautious in areas like the kitchen, break room, or bathrooms. Regularly clean and disinfect all surfaces in your work space and wash your hands before going back to work on your computer after breaking for a nosh. Use an EPA-registered disinfectant in the proper concentration, making sure it stays on the surface for a sufficient length of time to disinfect properly. You'll find this info on the product's label.

If a commercial disinfectant product is unavailable, you can clean and disinfect surfaces with a chlorine bleach solution (4 teaspoons of bleach added to 1 quart of warm water). Wearing gloves, dip a clean cloth in the solution and apply to surfaces until visibly wet. Let it go to work for 10 minutes, then rinse surfaces clean.

10 GERMIEST WORK SPACE PLACES

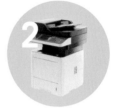

Surprise: most of them are not in the hardworking bathroom but other busy areas. Use extra caution where germs love to hang out.

1. Elevator Buttons

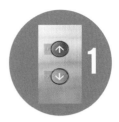

Your office elevator is probably one of the busiest places in the building. With a steady stream of hands pressing "lobby" or "parking" daily, the buttons are likely teeming with various germs. You could use your elbow to push the button, although you might get some funny looks. Always give your hands a quick wash with alcohol-based sanitizer after your ride.

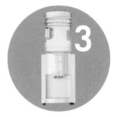

2. Office Equipment

Germs and bacteria thrive on the buttons and in the crevices of the busy printer, copier, fax machine, postage meter, and other high-tech office essentials. Sneezy Susie was here, after all. Put a tub of sanitizing wipes nearby to remind yourself to grab one every time you use a machine.

3. Watercooler

The office well is pretty popular in most offices. Germs can hitch a ride on bottles during transport and delivery. Eliminate any potential health risks by bringing your own water bottle.

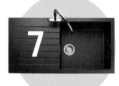

4. Coffee Maker

Bacteria can thrive and quickly multiply in the damp dark nether reaches of the office coffee maker. To sanitize, pour in 4 cups of plain white vinegar and let sit for a half hour. Run it through a brew cycle, followed by three more cycles of water, or until you don't smell the vinegar.

5. Coffeepot

If the coffee maker is a petri dish of germs, it's only natural that the coffeepot is less than hygienic. It should be washed thoroughly with warm soapy water after each use. Don't forget the coffeepot handle.

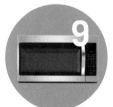

6. Coffee Mugs

One study found that 90 percent of office coffee mugs carried significant germs, including fecal matter. This is likely the result of coming into contact with germy sponges and dishcloths in a shared kitchen area.

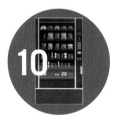

7. Sink

Just like at home, the sink is a magnet for bacteria. Clean and disinfect the sink regularly to keep germs to a minimum.

8. Kitchen Sponge

Sponges soak up and hold on to everything—that's why we use them. The warm moist surface is often home to disease-causing bacteria, including E. *coli* and *Salmonella*. So, every time we grab it for a quick surface wipe-down, we inadvertently spread germs all over the office (see #6 above). Disinfect daily (steps on page 85) and replace every two weeks.

9. Microwave Door

The microwave door handle is a hotbed of activity all day long as your coworkers zap lunch, mid-afternoon snacks, and coffee gone cold. All that touching leaves surface germs. Wipe all around and down the handle daily with a disinfecting wipe to keep germs in check.

10. Vending Machines

The buttons on about one in five vending machines tested in a large study were deemed likely to pass along illness-causing germs. While you could just swear off prepackaged food, an occasional wipe-down with a disinfecting wipe might be more effortless and protective enough.

BRINGING SAFETY HOME

Your home is your family's haven of safety, the place you return to each evening, leaving your worries (and the outside world) behind once you secure the door. But pathogenic germs can cling to the surface of items you carry in daily, like your busy debit card and the wallet it's in, your smartphone, and the keys that open that front door.

Always assume that whatever you bring into the house, or whatever you touch upon your arrival, is contaminated. I'm not being a pessimist here, just realistically protective. Upon return home each day, take a moment to wash your hands thoroughly and then clean and sanitize the items that came home with you.

Keyed Up

Face it: your keys are a cesspool. Giving your keys a bath in soap and water will wash away some of the surface germs, along with any dirt and grime. If you or someone who handles your keys was recently sick, however, the soap and water bath should be followed by the full disinfecting treatment.

Start by removing items like car remotes or decorative items that shouldn't get wet from the keychain. Mix a few drops of dish soap and warm water in a bowl, then swirl your keys around in the soapy solution.

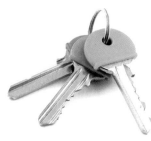

Use a brush to scrub away dirt and debris hiding in grooves and crevices. Swish in a bowl of clean water to remove the loosened gunk. Dry thoroughly with a clean cloth or rag. To sanitize and make sure no moisture is left behind (you don't want to risk rust), wipe your keys with a cotton ball dampened in isopropyl alcohol.

To go full out with disinfecting, use a disinfecting wipe or spray on all surfaces of your keys and keychain following label instructions.

Wallet Work

To de-germ a leather wallet (or bag), dip a microfiber cloth in warm water with a squirt or two of dishwashing liquid and blot-clean the leather. Dry with a clean towel. You can throw cloth wallets into the washing machine, then air- or tumble dry.

Clean Cards

One study found credit cards had more types of bacteria on them than cash and coins. To clean those germy cards, follow the steps on page 175. Make sure your card's magnetic strip and chip are completely dry before you slip it back in your wallet. If you're really concerned, consider using contactless payment options.

Sole Stuff

Turns out having a no-shoes-in-the-house policy isn't so extreme after all. A recent CDC report found illness-causing bacteria and infectious diseases could be living on your footwear. You don't have to let the freeloaders stay, however. First, remove all debris from the soles of the shoes with a toothbrush or shoe-cleaning brush.

Send mesh and canvas shoes for a spin in the washing machine in hot water with a product containing bleach if the fabric allows. Tumble dry on medium heat.

Clean leather shoes with a cotton or microfiber cloth dipped in cold water and a squirt of dishwashing liquid to remove visible dirt. Test an inconspicuous area.

To disinfect leather, dampen a clean microfiber cloth with 70 percent isopropyl alcohol. Test it on an inconspicuous spot on your shoes, then gently blot-clean the surface.

CLEAN CHOICES
Ditch Shoes at the Door

If you wear shoes at home now, it might be time to reconsider that decision. You could choose to make yours a shoe-free house and station a pair of comfy slippers by the entry door and change into them each time you come home. Not only will taking your shoes off by the door ensure that you won't be tracking dirt and germs into your home, but your floors and carpeting will stay clean longer, too. Try to slip shoes off simply with your feet, not engaging your hands.

GUESTS AND THEIR GERMS

Whenever friends or family visit your home, there is some risk of germs arriving with them. Right about now, you might be thinking, "This would be a good time to become a hermit." Yes, it would solve the immediate problem—keeping potentially disease-causing germs out of your home. But that would create a whole new set of problems—and the need for another book. Instead, shift into the "hostess with the mostess" mode and begin preparing your home and yourself for whatever shall come to pass. You're brave enough to open your home to friends and family—you've got this!

KEEP UP THE CLEAN ROUTINE. You can't eliminate the risk, but you can minimize it by preparing yourself and your home for the blur of activity and the dirt and germs likely to come with it. Keep up with the daily surface cleaning and disinfecting pre-visit, maintain that daily cleaning regime during the visit, and set aside ample time in your busy schedule for a thorough post-visit whole-house cleaning and disinfecting.

PLAN AHEAD. Counterintuitive though it may seem, plan for the unexpected by giving some thought as to how you'll safely handle the little surprises of life, such as receiving a hostess gift your guests will expect you to open right away. Should your visitors come bearing a gift, you might want to open the pretty box and discard the packaging outside your home, then wash your hands upon coming back inside.

CONGRATS!

Your Best Cleaning Resources & Next Steps

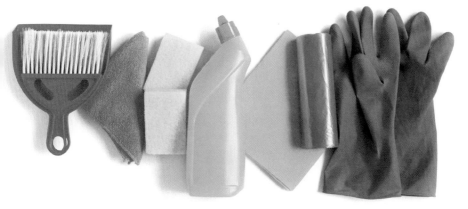

LIVING THROUGH A PANDEMIC opened our collective eyes to a nefarious new world of germs in our midst that we were suddenly called upon to conquer at home if we were to remain healthy. Some of these nasties, we learned, could be hitching rides on our shoes, purses, clothes, cell phones, and other previously novel surfaces (to us) in the realm of cleaning and disinfecting. Rather than panic (too much), we stepped up our cleaning game to meet the challenges.

At this point, fellow clean freaks and germaphobes, you're probably no longer tempted to dunk every germy thing you own in a vat of bleach. Now that you know how to sanitize every-thing in your home, you're well equipped to keep everyone in your home safe and healthy, come what may. You're safe to roam the world once more. Turn the page for a recap.

IN CHAPTER 1, you learned the critical difference between two words—*cleaning* and *disinfecting*—often used interchangeably. You know why doing one before the other is essential to eradicate the nasties. And, you learned how to safely execute this lethal one-two punch on surfaces throughout your home.

Germaphobes received the calming news that not all germs are out to put us six feet under. Exposure to some germs is good for us, as it helps strengthen our immune systems, leaving us better equipped to successfully battle harmful germs and stay healthy in the long run.

While you can't control every germ in your environment, it makes good sense to defend against the germs that can make you sick. You learned to hit germs where they live.

IN CHAPTER 2, you took a deep dive into high-touch surfaces in your home—light switches, doorknobs, and remote controls, the places viruses and bacteria inevitably set up shop. If left unchecked, these invisible interlopers can cause sickness ranging from the common cold and stomach bugs to food poisoning and vicious viruses. You learned how to focus your daily cleaning and disinfecting efforts on the "dirty dozen" germ hot spots.

IN CHAPTER 3, you learned how to sanitize hard nonporous surfaces in your home, including glass, metal, plastic, stainless steel, various countertops, tables and chairs, sinks, toilets, railings, light switch plates, doorknobs, and children's and pets' toys. These targets are especially important in light of a recent study that found the SARS-CoV-2 virus, which causes COVID-19, can cling to stainless steel and plastic surfaces for up to 72 hours, much longer than initially thought.

You also learned to clean and sanitize the most rigid surfaces of all in your home, the floors, including linoleum, vinyl, hardwood, laminates, stone, tile, and terrazzo.

IN CHAPTER 4, you took a walk on the soft side, learning how (and why) to sanitize soft surfaces in and around your home, including purses, backpacks and book bags, plush toys, carpeting, sofas and other upholstered items, area rugs, and shower curtains.

You discovered that while it is impossible to kill *all* microorganisms (disinfect) on soft nonwashable surfaces like carpets and upholstery, you can significantly reduce the level of bacterial contamination. Cleaning your cleaning tools—from mops, dusters, and brooms to the cleaning bucket and gross toilet brush—is now on your radar and easier than ever.

CHAPTER 5 took you into the once-mysterious world of sanitizing electronic devices, where you learned to sanitize the remote control and game controllers, your cell phone, computer, laptop, touchpads, keyboard, even your gross earbuds. After discovering how these devices' warmth encourages bacteria to multiply, you went forth, armed with safe sanitizing routines, and eradicated the teeming masses.

IN CHAPTER 6, you learned to disinfect your typical weekly laundry and the basket it rode to the machine in. You dug into how and when to disinfect the washing machine and the dryer, so they're always prepared to join in your germ battle.

IN CHAPTER 7, you navigated how to keep everyone in your home safe and healthy, while caring for an ill infectious family member. You learned how the daily disinfecting surface routine at home must undergo a shake-up when someone inside is sick, because some viruses can live on hard surfaces for up to two weeks. You also tackled how to remove sick stains on clothes—a tough job that you and your DIY solutions can now handle with ease.

IN CHAPTER 8, you traveled into public spaces filled with all sorts of bad bacteria—places like subways, airplanes, taxis, and public bathrooms—and held your own. You went to town on disinfecting groceries, takeout, packages, and mail. You picked up simple strategies for staying safe while out and about and smart ways to bring safety home. After all, pathogenic germs can hitch a ride on you or the many things you carry. You learned how to be smart about touching common surfaces like door handles, grocery store shopping carts, and restaurant menus.

You're now equipped with the knowledge of where germs lurk at home and in public spaces, and the methods and tools that can help keep them in check and your household well. Go forth, and be safe and healthy!

ACKNOWLEDGMENTS

A big thank-you to Chris Aronson Jr. for the OT editing assist from Brazil that helped make this book happen. It was indeed a joy to have you, my eldest son and fellow clean freak, back at home in the early months of the pandemic to help clean, sanitize, and redecorate the Santa Monica abode. I love you and am so proud of the upstanding young man you've become.

Thank you to my best friend, travel companion, and fellow night owl, Rose Ledger. Your friendship, support, sage advice, and sense of humor make roaming the world a never-ending series of memorable adventures! Your hubby, Steve, is right—you are my "sister from another mister." The only thing we don't share is a bloodline.

Thank you to Joseph Michael, my beach biking companion and personal trainer extraordinaire, for keeping me strong and on track. Your encouragement, support, and friendship these past few years have been invaluable. And to Joe Stuart Sarti, thank you for being a friend I can always count on to be there—through sickness and health. Your smile is infectious!

Thank you to Lori Musto, D.O., my physician and longtime friend, for being my go-to source on all things medical—and political. You're a beautiful walking encyclopedia of fun and knowledge!

My gratitude goes out to the whole team at Castle Point Publishing and St. Martin's Publishing Group for giving me a place to speak to and share strategies with households everywhere. Here's hoping we reach all those aiming for healthier homes!

I want to thank God most of all, because I wouldn't be able to do any of this without Him.

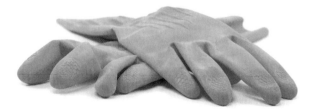

INDEX

brass, 52, 53
briefcases, 2
bronze, 52, 53
brooms, 82
buckets, cleaning, 83

C

cabinet knobs, 56–57
cabinets, wooden, 13
Campylobacter, 25, 43, 176
can openers, 54
carpets and rugs
    cleaning, 37, 68–70
    freshening powder for, 73
cars
    personal, 165–167
    ride shares, 168–169
car seats, 79–80
cash, 175
CDs, 103
cell phones, 17, 27–28, 90–94
Centers for Disease Control
    (CDC), 190
ceramic tile, 40
chairs, 31
checklists and cheat sheets
    daily cleaning, 32
    laundry room, 124, 136
    monthly cleaning, 39
    weekly cleaning, 37
chicken, safe handling of, 43
children
    hand sanitizer precaution,
        164

toys and equipment, 39,
    55–56, 78–81
chlorine bleach
    alternatives to, 121
    for cell phones, 92
    DIY disinfecting solution,
        12, 32
    expiration date, 13
    general use, 11–13
    for laundry, 133
    precautions, 13
chrome, 53
cleaning products and tools.
    See also disinfectants
    cleaning cloths, 22, 33, 63,
        85–86, 148
    gloves, 20, 33, 148, 155
    safety precautions, 21, 33
    storing, 22–23
    tool cleaning, 81–86
    2-in-1 cleaners, 11, 34
cleaning techniques. *See also*
    laundry techniques; *specific
    items or surfaces*
    daily cleaning, 27–32
    versus disinfecting, 8, 90–91
    hard surfaces, 49
    monthly cleaning, 38–39
    safety precautions, 32–33
    weekly cleaning, 34–37
clothes dryers, 122–123, 135
clothing. *See also* laundry
    techniques
    care labels, 128–130, 156
    germs on, 119

disinfectant for, 13
doormats, 69
doors, wooden, 13
drawer pulls, 13
dusters, 82
dusting
    during sickness, 152
    TVs, 105
dust mites, 44

E

earbuds, 112–116
E. coli
    disinfectant for, 133
    in kitchen, 43
    surfaces found on, 55, 56,
        79, 101, 176, 183
electronics
    cell phones, 90–94
    computer mouse, 100–101
    disinfectant for, 17
    DIY disinfectant for, 93
    fitness trackers, 111–112
    headphone cases, 116
    headphones and earbuds,
        112–116
    keyboards, 37, 95–96, 98–100
    laptop computers, 94–97
    remote controls, 31, 101–102
    during sickness, 150
    smart home devices,
        102–104
    smartwatches, 108–111
    speakers, 107–108

televisions, 104–107
elevator buttons, 181
Enterococcus, 74
enzyme detergent stain
    remover, 159
EPA (Environmental Protection
    Agency)
    disinfectant regulation, 8,
        10–11
    soft surface sanitizing
        products, 68
    website, 190
essential oils, antibacterial, 20

F

fabric softener
    alternative to, 122
    precautions, 86, 147
fans, 117
faucet handles
    daily cleaning, 29
    disinfectant for, 13
    in hotels, 172
fecal bacteria, 44
feces stains, 157
fels-naptha stain remover, 159
Fitbit guidelines, 112
fitness trackers, 111–112
floors
    carpeted, 68–70
    hard surfaces, 58–61
    weekly cleaning, 37
flu viruses
    disinfectant for, 133

stone floors, 60
stove knobs, 35
sunglasses, 166
supply caddies, 23

T

takeout dining, 179
taxis, 168–169
televisions, 104–107
terrazzo tile, 60
thermometers, 16, 141
tile
    bathroom, 40
    disinfectant for, 16
    floors, 61
toilet brushes, 84
toilets
    cleaning, 14, 30, 36, 63–64
    disinfectants for, 13, 16
    flushing, 61
    germ scale, 26
tools, disinfectant for, 16. *See
    also* cleaning products and
    tools
toothbrushes
    disinfectant for, 16
    sickness and, 152, 153
toothbrush holders, 36, 152
toothpaste, as chrome cleaner,
    53
touchless payment, 176, 179
touchpads, 56–57
touchscreens
    on airplanes, 171

cleaning, 17, 27–28, 90–94
towels
    bathroom, 36, 136
    kitchen, 36, 42–44, 136
    during sickness, 150, 153
toy boxes, 13
toys
    plastic, 39, 55–56
    plush, 79
train travel, 169–171
trash cans, indoor
    cleaning, 38, 65
    during sickness, 143,
        151–152
travel safety
    air or train travel, 169–171
    hotel stays, 171–172
    public transportation,
        167–168
    ride shares, 168–169
2-in-1 cleaners, 11, 34

U

ultraviolet (UV) light, 17
upholstery, 71–73
urine stains, 158

V

vacuum cleaners, 45
vending machines, 183
ventilation, 33, 152
vinegar
    for chrome, 53

as disinfectant, 17, 146
DIY cleaning spray, 8
general use, 17
for irons, 125
for laundry, 122, 134
vinyl floors, 58–59
vinyl tile, 40
viruses. *See specific viruses*
vodka, 14
vomit stains, 158

W

wallets, 184–185
walls, 61–62
washing machines, 39,
120–122, 156–157

wastebaskets
cleaning, 38, 65
during sickness, 143,
151–152
watercooler, 182
WD-40, as stain remover, 159
weekly cleaning, 34–37, 124
window cleaners. *See* glass
cleaners
wood floors, 59
wood furniture, 13
workplace surfaces, 180–183

Y

yeast, 55–56